Discovering Nutrition

Discovering Nutrition

Timothy Carr

Department of Nutritional Science and Dietetics,
University of Nebraska, Lincoln, USA

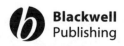
Blackwell
Publishing

© 2003 by Blackwell Science Ltd
a Blackwell Publishing company

350 Main Street, Malden, MA 02148-5018, USA
108 Cowley Road, Oxford OX4 1JF, UK
550 Swanston Street, Carlton South, Melbourne, Victoria 3053, Australia
Kurfürstendamm 57, 10707 Berlin, Germany

First published 2003 by Blackwell Science Ltd

Library of Congress Cataloging-in-Publication Data

Carr, Timothy P.
   Discovering nutrition / Timothy Carr.
     p.   cm.
Includes index.
   ISBN 0-632-04564-7
   1. Nutrition.   I. Title.
   QP141 .C28   2002
   613.2–dc21

ISBN 0-632-04564-7

A catalogue record for this title is available from the British Library.

Set in $10^1/_2$ on 12 pt Rotis Serif
by SNP Best-set Typesetter Ltd., Hong Kong
Printed and bound in
the United Kingdom by TJ International Ltd, Padstow, Cornwall.

For further information on
Blackwell Publishing, visit our website:
www.blackwellpublishing.com

Contents

Preface

Nutrition books come in two basic types; those written for consumers that cover the latest issues and hot topics, and university-level textbooks designed for in-depth, multi-year exploration of nutrition concepts. What seems to be missing is a book that offers a concise look at nutrition from the scientific point of view that is relevant to today's issues. This book was written to fill that void by serving as a resource for students, teachers, health care professionals, and consumers wishing to understand the full scope of nutrition in a concise and easy-to-read format. By eliminating much of the peripheral detail of a full textbook, the central topics of nutrition can be better emphasized. This book is well suited to students studying nutrition for the first time, as well as for health care professionals who wish to brush up on current nutrition issues and concepts. Consumers with a basic knowledge of biology will also find this book to be a valuable resource when making decisions about diet and health.

The general theme of the book focuses on the chemistry and metabolism of nutrients, and their impact on human health and well being. The chapters follow a logical sequence of the "life and times" of nutrients, from their presence in the environment (Part I) and the body (Part II), to their role in health and disease (Part III). The final section (Part IV) addresses many of the practical issues related to nutrition, such as choosing food wisely, interpreting nutrition information, and planning for a healthy future. Each chapter begins with a brief overview and ends with a "Chapter Test" that reviews some of the key points. You can "Check Your Performance" on the Chapter Tests to identify the topics that require further study. Additional review questions corresponding to each topic can be found in Appendix C. Each chapter also includes an "Application" of the chapter topic to real-life situations.

Few books are written in isolation, and several people have contributed greatly to this effort. I wish to thank Beverly Benes, PhD, RD, at the University of Nebraska for helping me realize the need for a fundamental nutrition review of this scope and for the many hours she invested during the planning stages. I also wish to thank Craig Hassel, PhD, at the University of Minnesota for his insights regarding "optimal health" and for helping me expand my view of nutrition beyond the scientific perspective. Many thanks also go to Ruth Rauscher, MA, RD, LMNT, for her knowledge of patient care and for encouraging me to emphasize the practical application of nutrition principles in everyday life. Her suggestions have helped make this book a useful resource for health care professionals.

Part I

Nutrients in the Environment

Chapter 1

Nutrition Discovered

Nutrition. The word can conjure up a host of images that mean different things to different people. Some people think of nutrition as a medical science in which biology, chemistry, and physics all play a role. Other people think of nutrition as a social or behavioral science that focuses on eating habits and factors that influence our food choices. Still others view nutrition from a global perspective, taking into account factors that affect food production and distribution worldwide. The full scope of nutrition, in fact, encompasses all of these perspectives, making it a truly multi-disciplinary field of study. And yet there is one common theme that ties each of these disciplines together: *the desire to better understand the interactions between food and living organisms.*

Essential Background

❖ Basic biology
❖ Basic knowledge about food and its availability

Topic 1.1

The Many Faces of Nutrition

> ### Key Points
>
> What is nutrition?
> What scientific disciplines contribute to the field of nutrition?

From the smallest bacteria to the mighty blue whale, all living things must receive a constant supply of food to sustain life. Despite this obvious fact, we seldom stop to think about all the different forms of food needed to sustain the many types of life found on earth. Every organism has evolved consuming the type of food to which it has best adapted. What may be a gourmet meal to a dung beetle may not be food to a honeybee. Even human populations have evolved consuming foods most readily available to them. Raw squid is commonly eaten in Japan; grubs are tasty treats for many Brazilian tribes; and Greenland Eskimos eat mostly seal and seabirds. It is quite remarkable how all forms of life, including humans, have adapted to their dietary surroundings in order to ensure the survival of their species.

The fact that living beings need food to survive is nothing new, but the notion that food contains specific "life-giving" substances—**nutrients**—is a fairly recent concept. The British physician James Lind (1716–1794) is generally credited with providing the first scientific evidence that certain foods—and, hence, specific nutrients—are needed to prevent ill health. In his now famous "A

Treatise of the Scurvy," Lind reported on his attempts to find a dietary cure for scurvy, a fatal disease common among sailors. We now know that scurvy is caused by vitamin C deficiency and its symptoms include bleeding gums, disorientation, and painful joints. Below is an excerpt from Lind's medical report:

I shall conclude the precepts relating to the preservation of seamen with showing the best means of obviating many inconveniences which attend long voyages and of removing the several causes productive of this mischief.

The following are the experiments.

On the 20th May, 1747, I took twelve patients in the scurvy on board the *Salisbury* at sea. Their cases were as similar as I could have them. They all in general had putrid gums, the spots and lassitude, with weakness of their knees. They lay together in one place, being a proper apartment for the sick in the fore-hold; and had one diet in common to all, viz., water gruel sweetened with sugar in the morning; fresh mutton broth often times for dinner; at other times puddings, boiled biscuit with sugar etc.; and for supper barley, raisins, rice and currants, sago and wine, or the like. Two of these were ordered each a quart of cyder a day. Two others took twenty five gutts of elixir vitriol three times a day upon an empty stomach, using a gargle strongly acidulated with it for their mouths. Two others took two spoonfuls of vinegar three times a day upon an empty stomach, having their gruels and their other food well acidulated with it, as also the gargle for the mouth. Two of the worst patients, with the tendons in the ham rigid (a symptom none the rest had) were put under a course of sea water. Of this they drank half a pint every day and sometimes more or less as it operated by way of gentle physic. Two others had each two oranges and one lemon given them every day. These they eat with greediness at different times upon an empty stomach. They continued but six days under this course, having consumed the quantity that could be spared. The two remaining patients took the bigness of a nutmeg three times a day of an electuray recommended by an hospital surgeon made of garlic, mustard seed, rad. raphan., balsam of Peru and gum myrrh, using for common drink barley water well acidulated with tamarinds, by a decoction of which, with the addition of cremor tartar, they were gently purged three or four times during the course.

The consequence was that the most sudden and visible good effects were perceived from the use of the oranges and lemons; one of those who had taken them being at the end of six days fit for duty. The spots were not indeed at that time quite off his body, nor his gums sound; but without any other medicine than a gargarism or elixir of vitriol he became quite healthy before we came into Plymouth, which was on the 16th June. The other was the best recovered of any in his condition, and being now deemed pretty well was appointed nurse to the rest of the sick . . .

As I shall have occasion elsewhere to take notice of the effects of other medicines in this disease, I shall here only observe that the result of all my experiments was that oranges and lemons were the most effectual remedies for this distemper at sea. I am apt to think oranges preferable to lemons, though it was principally oranges which so speedily and surprisingly recovered Lord Anson's people at the Island of Tinian, of which that noble, brave and experienced commander was so sensible that before he left the island one man was ordered on shore from each mess to lay in a stock of them for their future security . . . Perhaps one history more may suffice to put this out of doubt. (James Lind, London, 1753)

The work of Lind and other investigators helped lay the groundwork for the branch of science we now call nutrition. But the present-day study of human nutrition is much more complex because it involves more than finding foods (and nutrients) that prevent deficiency diseases. The full scope of nutrition encompasses the social, psychological, economic, and even spiritual influences that affect what we eat. It involves an understanding of chronic diseases and the implications of long-term dietary habits. The field of nutrition involves food scientists, geneticists, anthropologists, plant scientists, dietitians, psychologists, animal scientists, biologists, epidemiologists, clinical and laboratory researchers, pharmacists, and physicians. And in some cultures, nutrition is viewed from nonscientific perspectives, in which food contributes to the "balance" between the body, mind, and spirit. Thus, a thorough understanding of nutrition requires an awareness of many disciplines and perspectives, as well as the ability to interpret nutrition information in a technology driven world where the reliability of information is often highly questionable.

This book addresses the subject of nutrition largely from the scientific point of view. The primary goal is to provide an overview of nutrition that allows the reader to make well-informed lifestyle choices that promote good health and well being. The text emphasizes nutrient chemistry and metabolism, the role of nutrients in human health, and the many factors (internal and external) that challenge the healthful balance of nutrients.

Topic 1.2

Evolution of Nutrition Science

Key Points

How did the study of nutrition evolve into a science?
What key historical events contributed to our understanding of nutrition?

Nutrition entered the realm of science with the experiments of Sanctorius (1561–1636). Sanctorius, an Italian physician, published a report in which he weighed the amount of food and drink he consumed every day, then compared that to the weight of his excreta (feces and urine). He noted that his excreta weight was much less then the weight of his food and drink, yet his overall body weight did not change. He concluded that the weight of food and drink retained by the body was slowly lost as water through a process he called "insensible perspiration." Two centuries later, Lavoisier (1743–1794) conducted more refined experiments on the relationships between food intake and body heat loss, amount of oxygen inhaled, and amount of carbon dioxide exhaled. He concluded that heat produced by the body resulted from the combustion of food in a process that was similar to the process that takes place when substances are burned outside the body. From Lavoisier's work, we now know that the undetectable loss of food weight originally observed by Sanctorius was due to the loss of carbon dioxide through respiration, not perspiration (see Chapter 3). Lavoisier is often called the father of nutrition because the principles he established regarding respiration and metabolism are still used today. The experiments of Sanctorius and Lavoisier represent early milestones in nutrition that caused major shifts in thinking about the interactions between food and the body.

Another important milestone in the study of nutrition was the recognition that foods are made of specific components—**carbohydrate, protein,** and **fat**—that the body uses for energy. The French physiologist Magendie (1783–1855) was the first to distinguish between these three major nutrient categories. Liebig (1803–1873), a German physiologist, later showed that carbohydrate, protein, and fat were indeed the food components "burned" for fuel inside the body. He was also the first to estimate the energy content of foods. Although Liebig misinterpreted *how* the body uses carbohydrate, protein, and fat, he was correct in proposing that all three components are essential in the diet to maintain health.

In the late nineteenth century, several researchers attempted to reproduce milk in the laboratory using carbohydrate, protein, and fat isolated from cows' milk and other food sources. When the synthetic milk was fed to laboratory animals, they died. However, the animals survived if natural milk or other natural foods were added to their diets. This led to the conclusion that other vital substances must be present in food besides carbohydrate, protein, and fat.

Building on the research of Lind and others, the concept that deficiency diseases were caused by the lack of specific chemicals in the diet—and that consuming the chemical would cure the disease—was solidified by Cashmir Funk (1884–1967) and Frederick Hopkins (1861–1947) in their classic papers written in 1912. While Hopkins referred to these food chemicals as accessory factors, it was Funk who proposed the name vitamine—later shortened to **vitamin**—for these essential nutrients. The discovery and isolation of the vitamins dominated nutrition research in the early part of the twentieth century. Many students are surprised to learn that discovery of the vitamins is fairly recent, beginning with vitamin A in 1909. Vitamin B_{12} was not discovered until 1946. Even today experts are debating whether the chemical choline is an essential nutrient worthy of vitamin status.

The importance of dietary **minerals** also became apparent during the past century. The minerals needed in relatively large amounts (e.g., calcium and iron) were more easily studied and the first to be considered essential dietary components. Some trace minerals, however, are needed in very small amounts and were more difficult to study, especially when one considers the limitations of research methods in the early twentieth century. Although research methods used today are much more refined, the exact role of several trace minerals (e.g., boron and nickel) is still uncertain.

The past century was an exciting time for nutrition research, one in which nutrition was firmly establishing as an independent scientific discipline. The early studies have allowed us to view nutrition from a broad perspective in which every food substance we consume ultimately impacts our health and well being. Since the discovery of the vitamins and other essential nutrients, there has been a rapid decline in deficiency diseases among human populations. As we will see in later chapters, attention is now shifting from deficiency diseases to the role of nutrients in chronic diseases such as cancer, osteoporosis, and heart disease. The future of nutrition research will likely reach well beyond our traditional understanding of nutrients and, instead, focus on how substances in food can optimize health even in the absence of disease.

Topic 1.3

Definition of a Nutrient

Key Points

Why is there no single definition of a nutrient?
What do "essential" and "nonessential" mean?
Why is it sometimes difficult to distinguish between a nutrient and a drug?

Given the vital importance of food in sustaining life, nutrition researchers have for many years used the following definition of a nutrient: "Components of food that cannot be made in the body but are essential for normal growth and development." At first glance, this definition seems adequate and rather straightforward, as we know that the absence of essential nutrients will cause acute deficiency diseases leading to death. In fact, the discovery of the vitamins early in the twentieth century greatly reduced the incidence of several debilitating diseases such as scurvy, beriberi, and pellagra. However, the classic definition has become inadequate as we learn more about nutrients. Many issues regarding the nature of nutrients make it much more difficult to define them, and our simple definition is probably too narrow to cover the broad spectrum of what nutrients are and what they do. Most nutrition experts now recognize the limitations of the classic definition of a nutrient and are reluctant to create a simple one-size-fits-all definition.

Notice that the word **essential** is used in the classic definition, suggesting that a nutrient is something the body cannot make and is therefore required in the diet. Part of the difficulty in defining nutrients is that they may be viewed as substances in food that the body incorporates into its countless functions, whether or not those nutrients are made in the body. Cholesterol is an example of a food substance that the body uses for some very important functions, but humans do not need cholesterol in the diet because the body makes all that it needs. So while cholesterol is clearly not an *essential* nutrient, it can still be considered a nutrient because it is consumed in the diet and used by the body. Even more confusing are a handful of *essential* nutrients—including vitamin D—that the body makes, but the amount is usually too small to meet the body's needs. These nutrients are generally regarded as *essential*, even though they are occasionally made in amounts that satisfy the body's requirements. There are also examples of nutrients that can become essential if the body can no longer make them because of certain metabolic conditions. Cirrhosis of the liver and kidney dysfunction are examples in which the organs cannot make vital body chemicals, so dietary sources become important for survival. Premature infants also have difficulty making enough "nonessential" nutrients to meet the body requirements. Therefore, while the concept of essentiality is important, we must recognize that not all nutrients are essential and that some nutrients can become essential under certain metabolic conditions.

Nutrition experts currently recognize over 30 essential nutrients that humans require for normal growth, development, and the maintenance of health. There are probably dozens or perhaps hundreds more nonessential nutrients that the body uses even though there may be no absolute dietary requirement. A complete understanding of nutrients must therefore include their impact on long-term chronic diseases such as cancer, osteoporosis, and heart disease. Even some of the traditional nutrients known to be essential for the prevention of deficiency diseases are now thought to have biological effects on metabolic processes involving chronic diseases. Vitamin E, for example, has long been known to be essential for normal reproduction, although more recent evidence suggests it may also reduce the risk of coronary heart disease. This expanded role of the nutrients beyond the classic definition means that while some food substances are not essential for growth and development, their presence in the diet may help influence overall health and increase the quality of life. Nutrients that fall into this category include the many different chemicals naturally found in plants (phytochemicals). Nutrition researchers are just beginning to understand how these nonessential nutrients can help prevent chronic diseases and improve overall health and well being.

Given these considerations, no single definition of a nutrient can accurately summarize its full impact on human health and disease. It should be no surprise that most professional organizations such as the American Dietetic Association, the American Society for Nutritional Sciences, and the American Medical Association have avoided publishing nutrient definitions and, instead, strive to provide the general public with updated and accurate information that reflects our growing knowledge. It is also apparent that as we learn more, the line between "nutrient" and "drug" has become blurred. The legal definition of a drug is a substance that can treat, cure, and prevent disease—but so can nutrients naturally present in the food supply. Food companies are busy developing products enriched in some of these nutrients as a way of promoting health and preventing chronic diseases. The many roles of nutrients will be discussed throughout this book, including how essential and nonessential nutrients influence disease, as well as their impact on health in the absence of disease. The following section will provide a brief overview of the major *essential* nutrient classes and their functions. Other chapters will cover some nonessential nutrients and their role in promoting good health.

Topic 1.4

Overview of the Nutrient Classes

Key Points

What are the major nutrient classes and what do they do?
What are the major differences between macronutrients and micronutrients?
Why is water considered a major nutrient class?

The six essential nutrient classes are carbohydrates, proteins, fats, vitamins, minerals, and water. Each group may contain a variety of different substances, but all substances within each class share a basic chemistry or function that determines their classification. Carbohydrates, proteins, and fats are often referred to as the **macronutrients** because they are required in relatively large amounts in the diet. Another common feature of the macronutrients is their ability to provide the body with energy (see Chapter 3). Vitamins and minerals are considered to be the **micronutrients** because they are needed in only small amounts. Contrary to popular belief, the micronutrients do not contain energy and provide no energy to the body. However, some micronutrients participate in the chemical reactions that release energy from the macronutrients and are therefore essential for proper energy metabolism. Water is also an essential nutrient and, unlike the other nutrient classes, must be consumed daily to prevent water deficiency (dehydration).

Carbohydrates provide the bulk of most human diets and are the major sources of energy worldwide. Carbohydrates are a diverse family of substances that include **sugars**, **starch**, and **fiber**. Sugars and starch provide energy, whereas most dietary fiber provides no energy because it passes through the digestive tract and is not absorbed by the body. (A small proportion of fiber is metabolized by bacteria in the large intestine and, therefore, some energy can be captured for use in our bodies.) When we use the term "sugar," most people think of the refined white crystals commonly called "table" sugar. However, there are many types of sugars found in nature such as fruit sugar and milk sugar. Foods naturally rich in sugars include fruits, vegetables, honey, milk, and other dairy products. Sugar beets and sugar cane are particularly rich in sugar and are the major sources of commercially refined table sugar. Processed foods containing added sugars—such as candy and soft drinks—account for most of the sugar consumed in economically developed countries. Starch is found naturally in grains and vegetables, and is the primary carbohydrate consumed throughout the world. It is the main ingredient in foods such as beans, rice, potatoes, pasta, and breads. Refined starch is also used extensively in the food industry as a thickening agent in processed foods. Many people believe that eating foods containing starch and sugar are "fattening" and that sugar is more fattening than starch. In truth, starch and sugar provide exactly the same amount of energy, so sugar is no more fattening than starch. Furthermore, excess body fat is the result of consuming too much food, not just carbohydrates. Balancing the amount of food a person eats in relation to how much energy the body uses is discussed in Chapter 8. The term "fiber" refers to any plant material that is resistant to digestion and passes through the digestive tract unaltered. In this way, dietary fiber helps to prevent constipation and may lower the risk of colon cancer by speeding up the passage of fecal matter and substances in food that may cause cancer. One caution is that fiber in the intestinal tract may interfere with the absorption of other essential nutrients, although a well-balanced diet including plenty of fluids helps to ensure that all essential nutrients are consumed in adequate amounts.

Protein seems to have a more positive image than the other macronutrients. Unlike carbohydrates and fats, protein is usually associated with promoting good health and increasing one's strength and vitality. Athletes often choose high-protein foods or take protein supplements with the promise of increasing muscle mass, strength, and endurance. But does dietary protein deserve such a positive reputation? Does it really increase a person's strength and vitality? Should we be concerned about eating too much protein? A more complete understanding of what proteins are and what they do in the body is needed to accurately answer these questions. First, as an essential nutrient, protein is required in the diet to replace body proteins that are degraded as part of normal metabolism. Most people in developed countries consume about twice as much protein as the body needs. Second, the body uses only what it needs, so excess dietary protein is mostly "burned" for energy. Consuming excess protein does not automatically make muscles larger or become stronger—only exercise will do that! Finally, consuming high-protein diets does have some risks. The processing of protein in the body requires lots of water (about seven times more water than required for processing carbohydrates). Consequently, dehydration is a common problem, particularly for people who exercise and lose even more water through sweat and evaporation. Also, the kidneys are the only organs that can process the waste products of protein metabolism for elimination in the urine. An excess of dietary protein over time can overwhelm the kidneys and cause permanent damage. Like all nutrients, protein should be consumed as part of an overall balanced diet that contains adequate—but not excessive—amounts of protein. Overconsumption of protein can easily occur in economically developed countries where both animal and plant foods containing protein are readily available.

In contrast to protein, dietary **fats** have a negative reputation because of their link to heart disease and cancer. In some cases their negative reputation is justified, although the role of dietary fat in health and disease is very complicated and not fully understood by scientists. On the one hand, we know that certain types of fat are required for proper growth and maintenance of health, and their absence in the diet causes specific deficiency diseases. On the other hand, too much of certain kinds of fat can increase the risk of chronic disease. Part of the confusion is that several types of fat exist in nature and are present in the food we eat. Another point of confusion is that many different names are used to describe the substances in food we commonly call "fat." To a chemist, any molecule in food that does not dissolve in water belongs to a family of chemicals called **lipids**. The most important lipids in the food supply are **triglycerides** and **cholesterol**, which are chemically unrelated substances except for the fact that they do not dissolve in water. Triglycerides are the lipids commonly known as fat, oil, grease, shortening, lard, tallow, suet, ghee, and a variety of other names around the world. A bottle of soybean oil, for example, is pure triglyceride. We generally use the term "fat" to describe triglycerides that are solid at room temperature, and "oil" if they are liquid at room temperature. Fats and oils are actually mixtures of many different types of triglycerides with different chemical properties, which explains why some mixtures are solid and some are liquid. Triglycerides provide energy to the body and are found throughout the food supply in both animal and plant products. Cholesterol is another dietary lipid, but it is found only in animal products—cholesterol does not exist in the plant kingdom. You should be aware of clever marketing schemes that advertise plant foods as "cholesterol free" and then charge you a higher price! Cholesterol is made in the body in adequate amounts and is therefore not considered an essential nutrient. Unlike triglycerides, cholesterol provides no energy but it is a critical structural component of every cell in the body.

Mention the word **vitamin**, and an almost magical image comes to mind. Vitamins have been purported to do everything from boosting one's energy level to increasing sexual prowess to curing disease. While it is true that vitamins are required for a variety of metabolic functions, the restorative abilities attributed to them may be somewhat overstated. From the scientific viewpoint, vitamins are essential dietary substances needed in small amounts to regulate chemical reactions in the body. In this sense, vitamins are important for proper growth and maintenance of good health, but they appear to possess no greater properties beyond their basic chemical function. Vitamins do indeed participate in the chemical reactions that release energy from carbohydrates, proteins, and fats, but contain no inherent energy themselves. Vitamins are required for normal reproductive metabolism, but they are not aphrodisiacs. And inclusion of vitamins in the diet will cure disease, but only the specific deficiency diseases that develop in their absence. Vitamins are generally found throughout the food supply in developed countries and are consumed in adequate amounts, so despite popular belief, a vitamin supplement is usually not needed.

Minerals are among the basic elements of the earth that cannot be created or broken down by natural forces. Of the more than 100 earthly elements, the body requires at least 16 of them for a variety of functions such as conducting electricity, regulating chemical reactions, and providing structural components to the body. The minerals have traditionally been grouped according to the amount found in the human body or by how much is needed in the diet. The **major minerals** are those that comprise greater than 0.05% of total body weight, whereas the **trace minerals** are found in quantities less—usually *much* less—than 0.05% body weight. It is very likely that the body requires many more trace minerals than we currently believe, but they may be needed in such small amounts that current research methods are not sensitive enough to study their metabolic function. Minerals are generally found throughout the food supply. Plants obtain minerals from the soil in which they are grown, and animals accumulate minerals by eating the plants. Not surprisingly, the mineral content of foods is dependent on which minerals are present in the geographic region where the foods are produced. For example, there is a large region in China where the soil is deficient in selenium, and symptoms of selenium deficiency are common among the people that live in that region. Mineral deficiencies are rare in populations living in developed countries where the found supply is abundant.

Water is often the forgotten nutrient, yet it is the major component of our diet *and* our bodies. In fact, water is perhaps the most critical of all essential nutrients in the sense that humans survive only a few days without water, but can survive several weeks or months without other essential nutrients. The average adult consumes about 10 cups of water each day in the form of water-containing foods and beverages. While most water in the body comes from the diet, some water is generated from chemical reactions that occur during normal metabolism. Water is distributed throughout the body, both inside and outside cells. It provides several major functions in the body, such as lubricating joints, transporting nutrients in the blood, transporting waste products in the urine, regulating body temperature, and providing the medium for virtually every chemical reaction in the body. Physically active people require more water each day than inactive people because of increased water losses through sweat and evaporation.

Application

Humans depend on a constant supply of food for health and survival. Eating enough of the right foods in order to get all of the essential nutrients the body needs is not always easy to figure out, especially with the multitude of food choices available to consumers. To make matters even more confusing, health "experts" are continually warning us about foods we should avoid and which ones promote health. A few years ago consumers were told to stop eating butter because it caused heart disease and to switch to margarine. Then margarine became the bad guy because the type of fat used to make margarine was supposed to be worse than butter. This "good food/bad food" mentality has unfortunately created many misleading concepts and unfounded beliefs about food and its impact on health and disease. The nature of nutrition research is not black and white, and the apparently contrasting messages are merely a reflection of evolving knowledge and understanding of how nutrients function in the body. The first step in making healthy food choices is to realize there is no such thing as good foods or bad foods—all foods can fit into a healthy diet. In fact, no single food is perfectly balanced in all the essential nutrients required by the body. A healthy diet therefore depends on eating a variety of foods from several different sources, such as fruits, vegetables, meats, grains, milk and dairy products. This approach will help insure that all of the body's needs are met while helping to reduce the risk of chronic diseases.

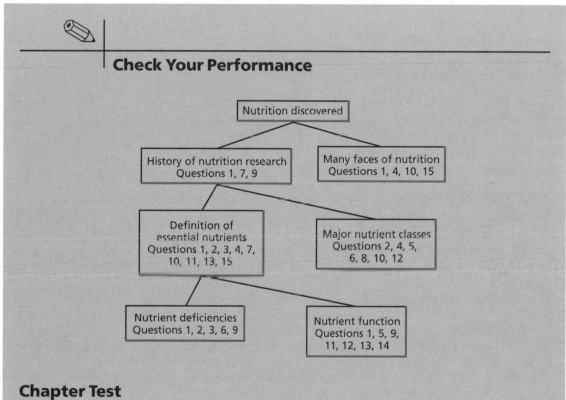

Check Your Performance

Chapter Test

True/False

1. All the essential nutrients needed for human growth and development have been discovered, and it is unlikely that new dietary substances important to nutrition will be discovered

2. Water is considered a nutrient even though it is not essential for growth and development

3. Certain substances in food can become "essential" nutrients if the body fails to make enough to meet requirements

4. Health and fitness magazines, such as *Prevention* or *Muscle*, are the best sources of scientific information for learning about nutrition and health

5. Certain nutrients are "burned" for energy in a manner similar to when substances are burned outside the body

Multiple Choice

6. Which nutrient class is most often associated with acute deficiency diseases?
   a. Lipids
   b. Vitamins
   c. Proteins
   d. Carbohydrates

7. Carbohydrate, proteins, and fats are considered macronutrients because
   a. They are more important than vitamins and minerals
   b. They are required in the diet in greater amounts than micronutrients
   c. They can be stored in the body
   d. They provide energy

8. Which of the following is *not* considered a source of dietary carbohydrate?
   a. Soybean oil
   b. Pasta
   c. Celery
   d. Table sugar

9. Some of the earliest studies in nutrition focused on
   a. Dietary fat and reducing the risk of heart disease
   b. Calcium deficiency and osteoporosis
   c. Curing scurvy with certain foods
   d. Reducing blood pressure by drinking milk

10. Which of the following statements regarding protein intake in economically developed countries is true?
   a. Protein is the most abundant nutrient class in the diet
   b. Protein supplements are usually needed to meet the body's requirement
   c. Animal foods provide the only source of dietary protein
   d. Protein consumption is twice the required amount needed by the body

Short Answer

11. Cholesterol is a vitally important component of every cell in the body. It is also consumed in the diet. So why is cholesterol not considered an essential nutrient?

12. Why are experts unsure about which trace minerals (and how many) are essential to humans?

13. What do vitamins do in the body?

14. Why is cancer considered a "chronic" disease?

Essay

15. Explain why a substance in food that is not absolutely essential for normal growth and development can still be considered a nutrient

Further Reading

Bidlack, W.R. (1996) Interrelationships of food, nutrition, diet and health: the National Association of State Universities and Land Grant Colleges White Paper. *Journal of the American College of Nutrition*, 15, 422–33.

Carpenter, K.J., Harper, A.E. & Olson, R.E. (1997) Experiments that changed nutritional thinking. *Journal of Nutrition*, **127**, 1017S–53S.

Center for Food and Nutrition Policy (1999) *What Is a Nutrient? Defining the Food–Drug Continuum* (M.L. Brown, ed). Georgetown University, Washington DC.

Olson, R.E. (1990) Evolution of nutrition research. In: *Present Knowledge in Nutrition*, 6th edn (M.E. Brown, ed.), pp. 502–5. International Life Sciences Institute, Washington DC.

Vanderbilt University Medical Center (1997) Nutrition History. (http://www.mc.vanderbilt.edu/biolib/hc/nutrition.html) Accessed 13 Jan 2002.

Chapter 2

Nutrients in Detail

The previous chapter provided a brief overview of the major nutrient classes and their basic functions. This chapter describes the nutrients in more detail, focusing on their unique properties and some of their major food sources. Information is provided about the nutrient characteristics that help us to better understand their function and what might happen when they are not present in the diet.

Essential Background

❖ Definition of a nutrient (Chapter 1)
❖ The nutrient classes and their primary functions (Chapter 1)

Topic 2.1

Carbohydrates

> ### Key Points
>
> What are the major carbohydrate classes and how are they related?
> What are the structural features of carbohydrates?
> Where are carbohydrates found in the food supply?

Carbohydrates provide the bulk of most human diets and are the major source of energy worldwide. The term carbohydrate literally means "carbon + water" and partially describes its chemical makeup. All carbohydrates contain carbon, hydrogen, and oxygen, and are typically found in a ratio of $1:2:1$, resulting in the chemical formula $(CH_2O)_n$. Carbohydrates are also called saccharides (from the Greek word "sakcharon" meaning sugar) and are usually divided into three groups: monosaccharides, disaccharides, and polysaccharides (figure 2.1). As their name implies, **monosaccharides** are simple carbohydrates comprising a single sugar unit. The most common monosaccharides are **glucose** ("blood sugar"), **fructose** ("fruit sugar"), and **galactose**. Note that glucose and galactose have nearly identical chemical structures, differing only at one point (indicated by arrow in figure 2.1). Fructose is found naturally in many fruits and vegetables and is the sweetest tasting monosaccharide. Food manufacturers have shifted to using high-fructose corn syrup as a sweetening agent because it is cheaper than regular table sugar and it has several functional properties that

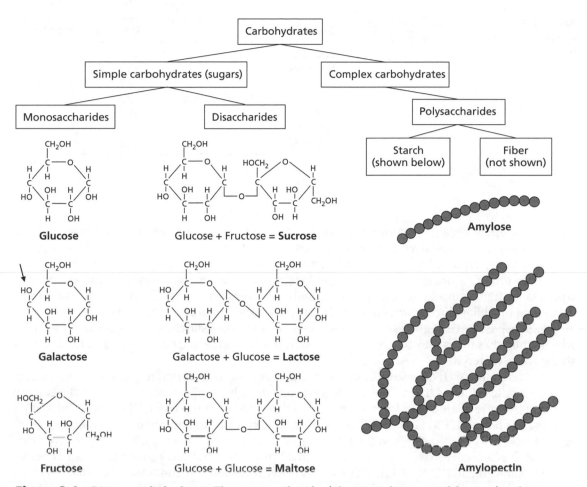

Figure 2.1 Dietary carbohydrates. The monosaccharides (glucose, galactose, and fructose) and disaccharides (sucrose, lactose, and maltose) comprise the simple carbohydrates, and the polysaccharides are referred to as complex carbohydrates. Digestible polysaccharides (starch) are found in nature as single chains of glucose (amylose) or as branched chains (amylopectin). The glucose molecules in starch are represented by the filled circles. Indigestible polysaccharides are referred to as dietary fiber.

are superior to table sugar. The soft drink and fruit drink industries are among the biggest users of high-fructose corn syrup.

Humans have had a "sweet tooth" for thousands of years. Ancient documents make clear reference to the use of honey as a sweetening agent. Sucrose (table sugar) became available only about a thousand years ago and has been the primary sweetener worldwide for most of the twentieth century. In addition, recent technological advances in food producing have allowed for the "invention" of another sweetening agent—high-fructose corn syrups (HFCS). The amount of HFCS consumed in the United States is now equal to sucrose and is found throughout the food supply in products such as carbonated and noncarbonated beverages, dairy products, canned fruits, jams and jellies, snack foods, desserts, breads, and a host of other baked goods. The development of HFCS and their introduction into the food supply is a good example of modern technology being applied to the benefit of society.

Food manufacturers became interested in fructose several years ago as an alternative

Table 2.1 Relative sweetness of several sugars and high-fructose corn syrups (HFCS)

Sweetener	Relative sweetness
Sucrose (table sugar)	100
Fructose	117
Glucose	67
50% fructose + 50% sucrose	128
HFCS-90	109
HFCS-55	99
HFCS-42	92

sweetening agent because fructose is the sweetest of all sugars commonly found in nature (table 2.1). Finding an inexpensive source of fructose, they reasoned, would allow them to replace sucrose and therefore reduce their production costs. However, while the monosaccharide form of fructose is found naturally in many fruits and vegetables, there are very few natural sources that would be available on a large scale (honey is one of the few exceptions). Eventually a process was developed in which glucose was converted to fructose using natural enzymes. All one needed was an inexpensive source of glucose—and that turned out to be corn starch. Starch from potatoes, rice, wheat, and other foods may be used, but corn starch is one of the most abundant and least expensive starting materials.

The production of HFCS results in 42% of the glucose being converted to fructose, which yields a product called HFCS-42. In order to make a syrup with higher proportions of fructose, the glucose and fructose syrups are separated, which yields a 95% glucose syrup and a HFCS containing 95% fructose. Blending HFCS-42 and HFCS-95 can provide syrups with intermediate amounts of fructose. Most applications in the food industry require HFCS containing 42, 55, 80, and 95% fructose. HFCS-55 has a relative sweetness nearly identical to sucrose and has proven to be an effective sucrose replacement. HFCS-55 is used extensively in the carbonated and noncarbonated beverage industry. A recent discovery that mixing fructose and sucrose improves their perceived sweetness (table 2.1) has allowed food manufacturers to reduce production costs by using less sweetening agent.

Disaccharides are also considered to be simple carbohydrates and are composed of two sugar units linked together by chemical bonds (figure 2.1). The disaccharides most important to nutrition are **sucrose** ("table sugar"), **lactose** ("milk sugar"), and **maltose** ("malt sugar"). Sucrose is formed in nature by combining glucose and fructose and is found in many plant foods. Other common food sources of sucrose are honey, maple syrup, and molasses (dark syrupy byproduct leftover from the sugar refining process). Sugar cane and sugar beets are the primary sources of commercially refined table sugar. Brown sugar and "raw" sugar are variations of sucrose available to consumers; brown sugar is made by mixing molasses with refined sucrose, whereas "raw" sugar is unrefined or partially refined sucrose. Of all the mono- and disaccharides, sucrose is the only one that can be called "sugar" on the ingredients list of food labels in the United States. Lactose is found only in milk and is formed in the lactating mammary gland by combining galactose and glucose. Maltose is two glucose units linked together and is found primarily in malted (germinated) grains such as barley. Maltose is found in products of the brewing industry and cereals made with malted grains.

Polysaccharides are classified as complex carbohydrates because they are composed of many sugars units linked together. The most important polysaccharides in nutrition are **starch** and **fiber**. Starch is composed of hundreds or thousands of glucose units linked together to form long chains (figure 2.1). A single long chain of glucose units is called **amylose**; when the glucose chain contains branch points it is called **amylopectin**. About three-fourths of starch found in nature is amylopectin. Starch is the main storage form of energy in plants that humans take advantage of, by harvesting the plants and incorporating the starchy foods into our diets. Some plants store starch above ground level in their seeds (e.g., beans, lentils, rice, corn, wheat), while others store starch underground in their roots and tubers (e.g., potatoes, yams, arrowroot, cassava, jicama). Although starch is easily digested, much of the remaining plant material is resistant to the human digestion. **Dietary fiber** is a collective term used to describe all nonstarch polysaccharides that cannot be digested. Dietary fiber is often further distinguished as **soluble** or **insoluble** fiber based on its ability to dissolve in water. In either case, indigestible fiber adds bulk to the diet and passes completely through the digestive tract in much the same form as when it entered.

Topic 2.2

Proteins

> **Key Points**
>
> What are the structural features of proteins?
> What are the symptoms of protein deficiency?

The word protein comes from the Greek word "protos" meaning "first" and was given by the Dutch chemist Mulder in 1838 to emphasize the importance of protein in human diets. Proteins are chains of **amino acids** linked together by a unique chemical bond called a peptide bond. There are 20 different amino acids that the body uses to synthesize proteins, nine of which must be obtained from the diet and are therefore called essential amino acids (table 2.2). The other 11 amino acids are made in the body and are called **nonessential** amino acids. If the diet is deficient in an essential amino acid, then body proteins that normally require that amino acid will not be synthesized even if adequate amounts of all the other amino acids are present. In this case, the one deficient amino acid is called the **limiting** amino acid. All amino acids are composed of carbon, hydrogen, oxygen, and nitrogen. The presence of nitrogen in the amino acids distinguishes proteins from

Essential amino acids	Nonessential amino acids
Histidine	Alanine
Isoleucine	Arginine
Leucine	Asparagine
Lysine	Aspartic acid
Methionine	Cysteine
Phenylalanine	Tyrosine
Threonine	Glutamic acid
Tryptophan	Glutamine
Valine	Glycine
	Proline
	Serine

Table 2.2 Essential and nonessential amino acids

carbohydrates and lipids, both of which lack nitrogen. Large proteins may contain several thousand amino acids in their chain, whereas small proteins may contain less than 100 amino acids. For example, insulin is an important regulatory protein in the body and contains only 51 amino acids. The unique properties of individual proteins are due to the length and specific arrangement of amino acids in the protein chain. Variations in the length and amino acid sequence allow for so many different proteins—with so many different functions—to exist in the body. However, just a single misplaced amino acid can cause a protein to lose its structural or functional properties, leading to metabolic disorders. For example, sickle cell anemia is a condition in which red blood cells cannot carry oxygen properly because one amino acid in the protein hemoglobin has been misplaced. In addition to transporting oxygen and other substances in the body, proteins provide structure to many tissues (e.g., bone and muscle proteins), they protect the body from foreign substances (e.g., skin proteins and antibodies), they regulate body functions (e.g., enzymes and protein hormones), and they help maintain fluid balance within the body's tissues.

Dietary proteins may be found in both plant and animal foods, and tend to be more abundant in the food supplies of developed countries. In developing countries, however, food supplies are often deficient in protein and total energy needed to support adequate growth and maintenance of good health. The result is **protein-energy malnutrition**. The term **marasmus** is given to the condition of severe muscle wasting and is primarily due to the lack of total energy in the diet. Occasionally, diets may be adequate in total energy (such as high starch diets) but lack adequate protein. The latter condition is called **kwashiorkor**, and its symptoms include dry skin and bloated bellies due to fluid accumulation in the abdomen. Kwashiorkor is a central African word meaning "the disease the first child gets when the second child is born." Symptoms of kwashiorkor develop when the first child is no longer breast-fed—displaced by the newborn child—and must begin eating the protein-deficient foods available in the community.

Topic 2.3

Lipids

Key Points

What are fatty acids and triglycerides, and how are they related?
What is meant by fatty acid "saturation"?
How is cholesterol different from fatty acids and triglycerides?

Lipids important in the study of nutrition are triglycerides and cholesterol. **Triglycerides** are the most abundant lipids in our food supply and are the main component of vegetable oils and animal fats. All triglycerides share the same basic chemical structure in which three **fatty acid** molecules are attached to one **glycerol** molecule (figure 2.2). When only two fatty acids are attached to glycerol, the chemical structure is called a diglyceride. One fatty acid attached to glycerol is called a monoglyceride. Mono- and diglycerides are rarely found naturally in the foods, but they are often added to high-fat "processed" foods such as margarine, shortening, and ice cream to help add smoothness and stability.

Figure 2.2 shows five different types of fatty acids: saturated, monounsaturated,

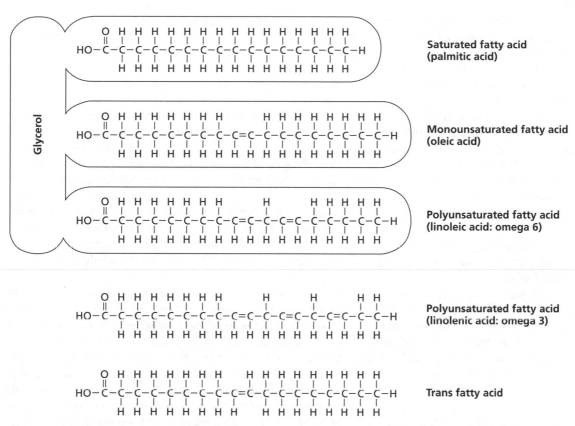

Figure 2.2 Dietary lipids. Three fatty acid molecules attached to a glycerol molecule comprise a triglyceride molecule (represented by the outlined area). When two fatty acids are attached, it is called a diglyceride; one fatty acid attached to glycerol is called a monoglyceride. Fatty acids are generally 16 or 18 carbons in length and may have varying degrees of hydrogen saturation. Linoleic acid and linolenic acid cannot be synthesized by humans and are therefore essential nutrients.

polyunsaturated (omega-6), polyunsaturated (omega-3), and trans fatty acids. Notice that when there are double bonds between carbon atoms, there are fewer hydrogen atoms attached to the carbon chain. When there are no double bonds, the fatty acid is fully **saturated** with hydrogen atoms. When one double bond exists in the fatty acid, it is **monounsaturated**, whereas a **poly-unsaturated** fatty acid contains two or more double bonds. Another way of describing fatty acids is the omega system. An **omega-6** fatty acid is one where the last double bond is six carbons from the end of the molecule (right side of figure 2.2); three carbons from the end is called an **omega-3** fatty acid. The degree of saturation is directly related to the physical properties of the fatty acid and, consequently, the triglyceride to which it is attached. Triglyceride mixtures that contain a higher proportion of saturated fatty acids tend to be solid at room temperature—for example, palm oil and beef tallow contain about 50% saturated fatty acids. Triglyceride mixtures that contain higher proportions of unsaturated fatty acids tend to be liquid at room temperature, such as soybean oil, which contains only about 15% saturated fatty acids. Chicken fat has an inter-mediate amount of saturated fatty acids (about 33%) and will become semi-liquid if left at room temperature.

The position of the hydrogen atoms on either side of the double bond is also an important feature that can influence the chemical properties of fatty acids. The vast majority of unsaturated fatty acids found in nature contain hydrogen atoms on the same side of the double bond. In chemistry this is called a **cis** double bond. Notice in figure 2.2 that the hydrogen atoms on both sides of the cis double bonds in oleic, linoleic, and linolenic acid are pointing down. When the hydrogen atoms exist on the opposite or transverse side of the double bond, the structure is called a **trans** fatty acid. Trans fatty acids exist naturally in the fat of ruminant animals (such as milk fat and beef tallow), although the majority of trans fatty acids consumed by humans come from **hydrogenated vegetable oils.** Hydrogenation is a process in which hydrogen gas is bubbled through liquid vegetable oil under pressure in order to increase the degree of saturation (i.e., decrease the number of double bonds). The longer the oil is exposed to hydrogen, the more saturated the fatty acids become, causing the oil to become increasingly more solid. Partial hydrogenation, while saturating some double bonds, can cause hydrogen atoms on some double bonds to shift into the trans configuration. The use of partially hydrogenated vegetable oils increased dramatically a few years ago as the use of animal fats in processed foods and restaurant cooking oils fell out of favor with consumers. The food industry relies heavily on hydrogenated vegetable oils for food products that must remain solid at room temperature. Products such as crackers, cookies, and pie crust simply don't work with liquid oils.

The impact of trans fatty acids on health has recently been called into question. The main concern is that dietary trans fatty acids tend to raise blood cholesterol levels and, therefore, may increase the risk of heart disease. A number of recent newspaper and magazine articles have further fueled public concern by suggesting that trans fatty acids are toxic to humans and that they create abnormal body chemistry. Like many nutrition and health issues, however, a great deal of unwarranted fear has been created. In fact, trans fatty acids are naturally present in both plant and animal foods, so they have always been a part of the human diet. The body metabolizes trans fatty acids just as easily as any other fatty acid that is absorbed from the diet, and no cases of toxicity have ever been reported in humans. And while trans fatty acids tend to raise blood cholesterol levels compared to monounsaturated and polyunsaturated fatty acids, they actually *lower* blood cholesterol levels compared to saturated fatty acids. In this regard, consuming foods that contain trans fatty acids in moderate amounts are safe and can easily be part of a balanced diet. The recent attention has prompted changes in food-labeling laws that will soon require the trans fatty acid content of foods be indicated on the label.

Describing fatty acids by degree of saturation or by the omega system is important in understanding how the different fatty acids function in the body. Humans lack the ability to make fatty acids with double bonds in the omega-6 or omega-3 position, yet these types of fatty acids are required for certain metabolic functions. Consequently, linoleic acid and linolenic acid must be consumed in the diet and are therefore **essential fatty acids.** The body converts these two fatty acids into a variety of other important chemicals required for growth and maintenance of health. Some people mistakenly believe that all dietary fat is bad and should be avoided at all cost. Essential fatty acid deficiency can result if linoleic acid and linolenic acid are absent in the diet. Fortunately, essential fatty acid deficiency is quite rare because the requirement is relatively small; there is enough linoleic acid and linolenic acid in 1–2 teaspoons (5–10 ml) of soybean oil, for example, to prevent deficiency.

Cholesterol is another dietary lipid important to nutrition, although its chemical structure and metabolic function are quite different from those of fatty acids and triglycerides. Cholesterol is a critical component of the body's cells and nerve tissue, and also serves as a building block molecule for the synthesis of vitamin D, bile acids, and steroid hormones. In fact the body can make all the cholesterol it needs for normal function, so cholesterol is not an essential nutrient. When cholesterol is consumed in the diet, the body adjusts by making less. A common misconception is that eating cholesterol automatically increases the amount of cholesterol in the body and, in particular, the levels of cholesterol in the blood. This is true only for about 15–20% of the human population who lack the ability to fully compensate for dietary cholesterol by decreasing the amount their body makes. For these people, a diet low in cholesterol is usually recommended to keep blood cholesterol levels from rising too high. Another important fact is that cholesterol is found only in animal foods; plants do not make cholesterol, so all plant foods are naturally "cholesterol free." A fun exercise is to look at the nutrition facts label of food products containing cholesterol and try to identify the ingredients that contribute cholesterol to the overall product.

Topic 2.4

Vitamins

Key Points

What do all the vitamins have in common and how do they differ?
What are some myths about vitamins?
Have all the vitamins been discovered?

All vitamins share a common function: they act as regulators of chemical reactions in the body. Table 2.3 lists the vitamins and their primary functions. The vitamins are generally grouped according to whether they dissolve in water or fat. An important distinguishing feature is that the **fat-soluble** vitamins can be stored in the body because they tend to accumulate in fatty tissues. By contrast, the **water-soluble** vitamins are easily excreted in the urine if not immediately used, so a relatively constant supply is needed to meet the body's requirements from day to day. (One exception is vitamin B_{12}, which has a longer "residence" time in the body than other water-soluble vitamins.) All of the water-soluble vitamins—except vitamin C—are also known as the "B" vitamins or

Table 2.3 Essential vitamins

	Primary function
Water soluble	
Thiamin	Helps release energy from macronutrients; promotes tissue growth
Riboflavin	Helps release energy from macronutrients; promotes tissue growth
Niacin	Helps release energy from macronutrients; promotes tissue growth
Pantothenic acid	Helps release energy from macronutrients
Vitamin B_6	Involved in protein synthesis; needed for red blood cell formation
Folate	Involved in protein synthesis; needed for DNA and RNA synthesis
Biotin	Involved in synthesis of glucose, protein, and fat
Vitamin B_{12}	Helps maintain nerve tissue
Vitamin C	Involved in collagen synthesis; acts as antioxidant
Fat soluble	
Vitamin A	Needed for proper vision; involved in cell growth and reproduction
Vitamin D	Needed for calcium absorption and maintenance of bone
Vitamin E	Acts as antioxidant
Vitamin K	Needed for blood clotting

the "B complex." Referring to them as a complex is somewhat misleading, because each is a distinct vitamin that exists independently from each other in the food supply. Some vitamins—vitamin B_{12}, vitamin D, and vitamin K—are actually made in the body, but the amount produced is too small to meet the body's needs, so they are still considered essential nutrients that are required in the diet. Furthermore, strict vegetarians who consume no animal products should be aware that vitamin B_{12} and vitamin D are found almost exclusively in animal foods and that a dietary supplement may be necessary.

Most people are aware of the importance of vitamins in maintaining good health. Since the mid twentieth century, nutrition education programs have helped consumers understand the role of a healthy diet in providing adequate amounts of vitamins and other nutrients. Unfortunately, this increased awareness has also created the concern—whether justified or not—that food alone might not supply sufficient amounts of vitamins. The vitamin supplement industry has capitalized on this concern and continues to promote the idea that vitamin supplements are necessary for good health. There are indeed situations where vitamin supplementation may be warranted (such as during pregnancy), although the majority of people living in developed countries where the food supply is abundant do not need to take a vitamin supplement. The practice of consuming vitamin supplements is costly and can easily lead to misuse and overconsumption (see Chapter 4). One should always check with a physician, registered dietitian, or other qualified health care professional before taking vitamin supplements.

Another important chemical that functions in the human body is **choline**. It deserves special mention because the National Academy of Sciences has recently recommended that choline be given essential nutrient status. Like some vitamins, choline is made in the body but may not be made in high enough amounts to meet the body's requirement. Some studies have shown that humans, particularly males, can become deficient in choline if dietary sources are removed. Much more research will be needed before recommended levels of dietary choline are established.

In addition to the current list of vitamins, there exists a wide variety of nonessential substances that enter our bodies when we consume food. While not absolutely required for survival, these substances can influence the body's metabolism and thus impact overall health. Scientists have begun to examine a group of substances called **phytochemicals**. The term phytochemical is based on the Greek word "phyto" meaning "plant," and refers to the hundreds of substances found in plant foods (see Chapter 13). Certain phytochemicals are believed to reduce the risk of heart disease, cancer, hypertension, stroke, diabetes, and a variety of other disorders, although how they work in the body is not completely understood.

Consumers should also be aware of **bogus vitamins**—substances that are not required in diet or have absolutely no function in the body. Because of the mystery that often surrounds the purported health benefits of vitamins, unscrupulous manufacturers and marketers have created a multi-billion dollar industry that preys on the public's lack of awareness in nutrition and how the body functions. A brief list of these substances includes coenzyme Q_{10}, carnitine, lipoic acid, PABA, laetrile (sometimes called vitamin B_{17}), pangamic acid (sometimes called vitamin B_{15}), and rutin and hesperidin (both sometimes called vitamin P). What may be confusing for some people is that many of these substances are indeed present in the body and do provide important functions. However, in every case the body makes ample amounts, and studies have not been able to show that removal of any one of these substances from the diet produces deficiency diseases.

Topic 2.5

Minerals

Key Points

To what extent are the major minerals and trace minerals different?
What are the electrolytes?
What common disorders result from mineral deficiency?

Minerals are among the basic elements of the earth that cannot be created or broken down by natural forces. Of the more than 100 earthly elements, the body requires at least 16 of them for a variety of functions such as conducting electricity, regulating chemical reactions, and providing structural components to the body. Table 2.4 lists the essential minerals and their primary functions. The minerals have traditionally been grouped according to the amount found in the human body. The **major minerals** are those that comprise greater than 0.05% of total body weight, whereas the **trace minerals** are found in quantities less—usually *much* less—than 0.05% body weight. It is very likely that the body requires many more trace minerals than those listed in table 2.4, but they may be needed in such small amounts that current research methods are not sensitive enough to study their metabolic function.

A special group of minerals called **electrolytes** include sodium, potassium, and chloride. As their name suggests, these minerals function in electrical reactions that control nerve conduction and muscle contraction. Because they have an electrical charge when dissolved in body fluids, they help

Table 2.4 Essential minerals

Mineral	Primary function
Major minerals	
Sodium	Regulates water balance in body tissues; needed for nerve conduction
Potassium	Regulates water balance in body tissues; needed for nerve conduction
Chloride	Regulates water balance in body tissues
Calcium	Structural component of bone and teeth; needed for nerve conduction
Phosphorus	Structural component of bone and teeth
Magnesium	Structural component of bone and teeth; activates enzymes
Sulfur	Part of amino acids and vitamins
Trace minerals	
Iron	Transports oxygen as part of hemoglobin, red blood cells
Copper	Activates enzymes involved in many body systems
Zinc	Activates enzymes involved in growth and development
Manganese	Needed for carbohydrate and lipid metabolism
Selenium	Acts as antioxidant
Iodine	Needed for synthesis of thyroid hormones
Chromium	Needed for glucose metabolism
Fluoride	Component of bone and teeth
Molybdenum	Activates enzymes involved in many body systems

to regulate fluid balance and blood pressure (hypertension). Some studies have suggested that too much sodium in the diet can cause a fluid imbalance that results in elevated blood pressure, prompting many health organizations to recommend limiting sodium intake. At first glance, this recommendation seems rather straightforward, but it is not without controversy. Disagreement regarding the usefulness of the recommendation stems from the fact that only a small proportion (10–15%) of the human population is "salt sensitive"—that is, their blood pressure changes in response to the amount of sodium they consume. That means that blood pressure in most people (85–90% of the population) is unaffected by dietary sodium. While public health officials acknowledge these statistics, they still believe that providing population-wide recommendations is the best approach so that those individuals most at risk will benefit. The evidence that other factors besides dietary sodium contribute to high blood pressure adds to the controversy. One approach for individuals with high blood pressure is to try limiting their salt and sodium intake to see if their blood pressure goes down. If so, then they could benefit from a salt-restricted diet. If blood pressure does not decrease on a salt-restricted diet, then other factors are involved and these may require medical intervention.

Deficiencies of several minerals are fairly common even in developed countries. Insufficient calcium, iron, and iodine are examples of dietary minerals that produce well-defined deficiency diseases. Calcium is important in bone formation where it binds with phosphorus to form a rigid crystalline structure called hydroxyapatite. Insufficient calcium during early bone development can lead to reduced bone mass and **osteoporosis** later in life (see Chapter 9). Iron is a vital component of hemoglobin, which in found in red blood cells and is responsible for carrying oxygen in the blood. When iron is in short supply, hemoglobin cannot be made and the number of red blood cells decreases. The result is **iron deficiency anemia,** in which too few red blood cells are unable to deliver enough oxygen to tissues. The symptoms of iron deficiency anemia are consistent with the function of iron in red blood cells and include fatigue and headache. Most of the iodine in the environment is found in the sea, so the best dietary sources are seafood and plants grown near or in the ocean. Not surprisingly, iodine deficiency is most common in parts of the world that are far removed from the ocean. Because iodine is needed for synthesis of thyroid hormones, iodine deficiency results in enlargement of the thyroid gland (called a **goiter)** located in the neck just above the sternum. Iodine deficiency during pregnancy can affect fetal development, resulting in mental retardation of the child, spontaneous abortions, and stillbirths. Many countries have addressed iodine deficiency by adding iodine to their salt supplies.

Topic 2.6

Water

Key Points

What is meant by "water balance"?
What happens when the body becomes dehydrated?

Water is often the forgotten nutrient, yet it is the major component of our diet *and* our bodies. The average adult consumes about 10 cups of water each day in the form of water-containing foods and beverages. To maintain **water balance**, this means that the same person needs to eliminate 10 cups of water each day through urinary and fecal output, and through evaporation from the skin and lungs (known as insensible water loss). While most water in the body comes from the diet, a small proportion is generated from chemical reactions that occur during normal metabolism. Water provides several major functions in the body, such as lubricating joints, transporting nutrients in the blood, transporting waste products in the urine, regulating body temperature, and providing the medium for virtually every chemical reaction in the body.

The amount of **body water** is highly regulated and humans can survive only a few days without replacing lost body water. The loss of just 2–3% body water can cause **dehydration** and a decrease in blood volume, so that oxygen and nutrient transport is compromised. A loss of 5% causes mental confusion and disorientation, and a loss of 10% can cause death. Athletes and people who perform strenuous work need to consume large amounts of water—perhaps even when they do not feel thirsty—to replace body water lost through sweat and respiration. Prolonged episodes of diarrhea, vomiting, fever, and exposure to hot weather can increase the demand for water. Consumption of high-protein diets also increases the need for water because protein metabolism uses body water for processing. Caffeine and alcohol are diuretics (they increase urine output), therefore their consumption increases demand for water.

Most foods and beverages contain water—even butter contains water. Milk is about 90% water, most fruits and vegetables about 80%, eggs about 70%, and meat about 60%. Two-thirds of our dietary water comes from beverages and one-third from foods, so even though foods contain water, it is important to drink about six cups of water as beverages every day. In some parts of the world, however, fresh drinking water is not always available. Water shortages due to drought, pollution, overuse and misuse are increasing concerns about whether there will be enough fresh water for the twenty-first century. There is clearly a need for better water management programs worldwide to ensure enough fresh water for agriculture and personal consumption. Concerns about the safety of municipal water supplies have prompted many people to support the multi-billion dollar bottled water industry. Contrary to popular belief, bottled water may be no better than tap water with regard to health and safety. Bottled water does have the advantage of being packaged in convenient personal-sized containers, and it may even taste better than tap water. However, the Food and Drug Administration, which regulates the bottled water industry in the United States, estimates that 25% of the bottled water sold in the United States actually comes from municipal water supplies. Regardless of the source, the FDA requires that all bottled water sold in the United States conform to minimum standards of quality and not exceed the allowable levels of chemical contaminants in their products.

Application

Constipation is a common problem among people of all ages and is generally defined as "the infrequent and difficult elimination of feces." One of the best ways to treat constipation is to increase the consumption of dietary fiber and fluids on a regular basis. The primary effect of dietary fiber on bowel function is attributed to its water-holding capacity. Both soluble and insoluble fiber can bind water, which softens the feces and increases its bulk, making it easier to eliminate. Because dietary fiber draws body water into the bowel, increases in fluid intake must accompanying increases in fiber intake or dehydration can occur. Both constipation and dehydration are common problems among the elderly. Older adults tend to lose their ability to taste and smell, so food consumption—including foods rich in dietary fiber—decreases. They also tend to lose sensitivity in their brain's thirst sensors, so fluid intake is often inadequate to maintain a healthy fluid balance. Older adults are often advised to drink fluids throughout the day even when they do not feel thirsty in order to prevent dehydration. Adopting a diet that includes high-fiber foods and increased fluids is the safest way to prevent constipation, but it is estimated that 20–30% of people over age 65 are dependent on laxatives as a treatment for constipation.

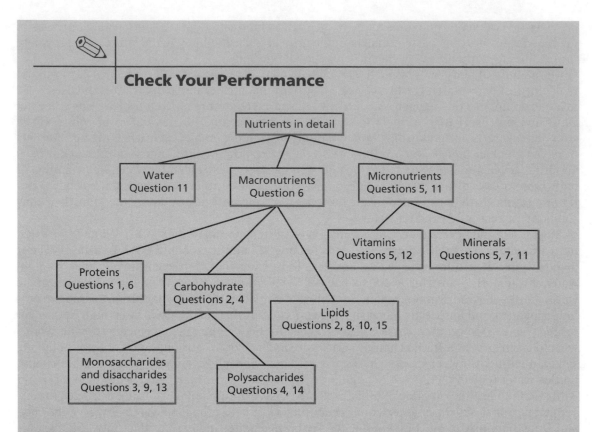

Check Your Performance

Chapter Test

True/False
1. All proteins, regardless of their size, are made from 20 different amino acids
2. Triglycerides are the most abundant nutrients in the human diet worldwide
3. Eggs are a major source of lactose in the diet
4. The term "complex carbohydrates" refers to dietary polysaccharides
5. Nerve conduction and muscle contraction are the primary functions of the trace minerals

Multiple Choice
6. Which of the following criteria distinguishes proteins from carbohydrates and lipids?
    a. Proteins may be used for energy
    b. Insufficient dietary protein causes deficiency diseases
    c. Proteins contain nitrogen
    d. Proteins are required in the diet
7. Besides salt added to food at the table, the most likely source of sodium in the food supply is
    a. Fresh meats
    b. Packaged and canned foods
    c. Marine foods (fish, shellfish, etc.)
    d. Fresh vegetables

8. Which of the following foods contain cholesterol?
   a. Peanut butter
   b. Vegetable shortening
   c. Sour cream
   d. Margarine
9. Major sources of fructose in the diet include
   a. Fruits and vegetables
   b. Wheat flour
   c. Milk and cheese
   d. Soybeans
10. Fats and oils become more solid at room temperature by increasing the amount of
    a. Mono- and diglycerides
    b. Double bonds
    c. Polyunsaturated fatty acids
    d. Saturated fatty acids

Short Answer

11. Minerals are often lost from the body through sweat. If you worked for a food company that made sports drinks, what would be the most likely minerals you would add to your product as a way of replacing those lost through sweat?
12. Which vitamins are likely to be most toxic if consumed in excess amounts for a long period of time?
13. Describe which monosaccharides (and their primary ingredient source) you would be ingesting if you ate a milk chocolate candy bar
14. What is dietary fiber?

Essay

15. What are trans fatty acids and what is their effect on health?

Further Reading

Ames, B.N. (1999) Micronutrient deficiencies. A major cause of DNA damage. *Annals of the New York Academy of Sciences*, **889**, 87–106.

Duffy, V.B. & Anderson, G.H. (1998) Position of the American Dietetic Association: use of nutritive and non-nutritive sweeteners. *Journal of the American Dietetic Association*, **98**, 580–7.

Giboney, M., Sigmann-Grant, M., Stanton, J.L. & Keast, D.R. (1995) Consumption of sugars. *American Journal of Clinical Nutrition*, **62**(Suppl.), 178S–94S.

Mertz, W. (1998) Review of the scientific basis for establishing the essentiality of trace elements. *Biological Trace Element Research*, **66**, 185–91.

Popkin, B.M., Siega-Riz, A.M., Haines, P.S. & Jahns, L. (2001) Where's the fat? Trends in US diets 1965–1996. *Preventive Medicine*, **32**, 245–54.

Reeds, P.J. (2000) Dispensable and indispensable amino acids for humans. *Journal of Nutrition*, **130**, 1835S–40S.

Vuilleumier, S. (1993) Worldwide production of high-fructose syrup and crystalline fructose. *American Journal of Clinical Nutrition*, 58(Suppl. 5), 733S–6S.

Yates, A.A., Schlicker, S.A. & Suitor, C.W. (1998) Dietary Reference Intakes: the new basis for recommendations for calcium and related nutrients, B vitamins, and choline. *Journal of the American Dietetic Association*, 98, 699–706.

Chapter 3

The Circle of Life

All life on earth depends on a constant supply of energy. Humans are able to capture energy from the environment by eating food that contains energy. Remarkably, all of the energy that is present on earth can be traced to a single source—the sun. Plants use the sun's energy to make carbohydrates and other essential nutrients that may be consumed by humans or by grazing animals, which are then consumed by humans. The process of transferring energy from the sun to the human body involves the constant building and breaking down of molecules that have the ability to hold energy so that it may be transferred from one biological system to another. The macronutrients—carbohydrates, proteins, and lipids—are examples of molecules that can hold the sun's energy for use by humans and other animals. This chapter will focus on how carbon, hydrogen, and oxygen atoms are continually arranged and rearranged into various molecules during the transfer of energy. In this sense, molecules are constantly being transformed and shuttled between plants and animals as part of a giant recycling program that is essential for life.

Essential Background

- ❖ Basic chemical makeup of the nutrient classes (Chapter 2)
- ❖ Biological relationship between plants and animals
- ❖ Concept of the "food chain"

Topic 3.1

Energy—Universal Life Support

> **Key Points**
>
> What is energy?
> Where does energy come from?
> How is energy measured?

Energy is a fascinating phenomenon of nature. We all seem to have a general understanding of what it is, but defining it is not so easy because energy can come in many different forms such as **heat** energy, **electrical** energy, **light** energy, and **mechanical** energy. The traditional definition of energy is quite broad and is usually stated as "the ability to do work." An example of heat energy performing work is a hot air balloon, which can lift considerable weight against the force of gravity simply because the air inside the balloon is hotter than the surrounding environment. A lightning strike can split a tree in half with pure electrical energy. Physicians who use lasers during surgery are making use of light energy to perform work. And a rock falling down a hillside can produce a tremendous amount of mechanical energy, particularly if you are standing in its path! Each form of energy—heat, electrical, light, and mechanical—is present inside the human body and performs some sort of work. Nutrition researchers are mostly concerned with how energy in food is captured and used by the body for processes such as muscle movement, synthesizing vital molecules, and transferring genetic information.

All of the energy present in the food supply ultimately comes from the sun. Through a complex process called **photosynthesis**, plants are able to synthesize carbohydrates using light energy. Recall that most carbohydrates are composed of carbon, hydrogen, and oxygen in the proportion of $1:2:1$ $(CH_2O)_n$. In making carbohydrates, plants are able to combine carbon dioxide (CO_2) from the atmosphere with water (H_2O) from the soil. The process releases oxygen (O_2) into the atmosphere as a "waste" product that animals and other organisms use for normal metabolism. The overall chemical reaction of photosynthesis can be written as:

$$CO_2 + H_2O + \text{Light Energy} \rightarrow \text{Carbohydrate} + O_2$$

Starch and sucrose are the major carbohydrates made during photosynthesis, which then serve as important sources of energy for the plant to make amino acids (for protein) and fatty acids (for triglyceride) during its normal growth. Grazing animals obtain their energy by feeding on the plants, while predatory animals feed on grazing animals. A similar chain of events occurs in the ocean, where marine plants—mostly microscopic in size—use photosynthesis to convert CO_2 and H_2O into carbohydrates. These marine plants are eaten by small marine herbivores, which in turn are eaten by larger carnivores, and so on. Humans benefit from being at the end of the "food chain" by having available to us all of these different foods and energy sources. In this way, the presence of energy in virtually every biological system is completely dependent on the ability of plants to capture light energy from the sun and convert it into forms that other living organisms can use. Without question, photosynthesis is the most critical biochemical process on earth because it is the only way that living systems are able to harness energy from an external source.

The amount of energy in food—and therefore the amount of energy available to the body—can be measured by relatively simple methods. The most common technique takes advantage of the fact that when something is burned in the presence of oxygen it gives off heat. When foods are burned (or oxidized), the amount of heat energy given off represents the total amount of energy present in the food. The unit of measurement for heat energy is the **calorie**, defined as the amount of heat required to raise the temperature of 1 gram of water 1°C. The amount of energy in one calorie is actually quite small relative to how much energy people consume each day. Consequently, nutrition professionals usually deal with 1,000-calorie increments, expressed as a **kilocalorie, kcalorie, kcal,** or **Calorie** with a capital "C." Energy information found on food labels is always written as Calories. The amount of energy in food can also be estimated if you know how much carbohydrate, protein, and fat is in the food. Carbohydrates and proteins provide 4 kcal per gram, whereas fat provides 9 kcal per gram. Therefore, a blueberry muffin that contains 20 grams of carbohydrate, 2 grams of protein, and 3 grams of fat will provide 115 kcalories:

(20 grams carbohydrate $\times$ 4 kcal/g) + (2 grams protein $\times$ 4 kcal/g) + 3 grams fat $\times$ 9 kcal/g) =
   (80 kcal from carbohydrate) + (8 kcal from protein) + (27 kcal from fat) = 115 total kcalories

Alcohol is another substance in the food supply that provides energy (7 kcal per gram), although there is some debate among health professionals whether alcohol should be considered a nutrient. Alcoholic beverage has been used both socially and medicinally for thousands of years, but history has shown that it can be both harmful and beneficial to health. Moderate drinkers have a lower incidence of heart disease, stroke, and high blood pressure than nondrinkers—and they live longer than nondrinkers! The health benefits of alcohol are illustrated by a situation known as the "French Paradox." Among 18 economically developed countries (including the United States), France has the lowest mortality rate, yet saturated fat intake, plasma cholesterol levels, and blood pressure are not lower than that of other countries. One difference is that the French are the leading consumers of wine in the world. While there are clearly other lifestyle and environmental difference among developed countries, many consumers in the United States have followed suit by drinking a glass of wine each day to "keep the heart healthy." Even the United States government and the American Heart Association have acknowledged that moderate drinking can help people live longer. The American College of Cardiology has approached it from a different angle by citing the avoidance of alcohol as *increasing* the risk for heart disease.

However, overconsumption can lead to heart disease, hemorrhagic stroke, high blood pressure, liver disease, nutrient deficiencies, brain dysfunction, and premature death. Alcoholism also contributes to a host of psychological and social problems. When considering alcohol consumption, several issues need to be considered:

What constitutes "moderate" drinking? In 1995, the US Dietary Guidelines Advisory Committee defined moderate alcohol intake as less than or equal to one drink a day for women and less than or equal to two drinks a day for men. One drink was defined as one 12-ounce glass of beer, one 5-ounce glass of wine, or one 1.5-ounce "shot" of 80-proof distilled spirits. Some studies suggest that even less—perhaps two or three drinks per week—can be effective at helping reduce the risk of chronic disease compared to not drinking at all.

Who might benefit and might not? Research suggests that men over the age of 40 and postmenopausal women are those most likely to benefit from moderate alcohol consumption. Men under 40 years are generally not at risk for heart disease and other chronic diseases for which moderate drinking is thought to be beneficial. Moreover, most alcohol-related accidents and acts of violence involve men under 40 years of age, so promoting drinking in this age group seems to be socially irresponsible. With regard to women, the benefits of moderate alcohol consumption would only be realized after menopause when their risk of heart disease and stroke increases due to declining estrogen levels. Because the risk for these diseases is lowest prior to menopause, moderate drinking in younger women offers no real health benefits. On the contrary, alcohol consumption during pregnancy greatly increases the risk of birth defects, so abstaining from alcohol is the best health strategy for women who wish to become pregnant.

Should nondrinkers start drinking? It's important to consider all of the reasons why people decide not to drink. Often a person's decision to abstain is based on religious, social, and personal concerns that are not necessarily related to health. Nondrinkers should not feel pressured into drinking with the belief that alcohol will automatically produce health benefits. A full understanding of the potential risks and benefits must be taken into account, as well as the added responsibility that goes along with consuming alcohol. And as with most nutrition and health issues, the benefits gained from any dietary change will vary among individuals so that not everyone will realize the benefits of moderate drinking.

Topic 3.2

Nutrient Recycling

Key Points

What is an organic molecule?
In what forms are carbon, hydrogen, oxygen, and nitrogen recycled between plants and animals?
How are minerals recycled between plants and animals?

All of the earth's biological systems depend on each other for nutrients. There exists a great sharing of resources—a recycling of sorts—that must remain in constant balance if all living things are to survive. At the core of this nutrient recycling is the exchange of **carbon** atoms that occurs between plants and animals (figure 3.1). Carbon is shuttled from humans and other animals back to plants in the form of carbon dioxide (CO_2) so that plants can make carbohydrates and other **organic** molecules such as proteins, lipids, and vitamins. (In science, the term "organic" refers to the chemistry of carbon and should not be confused with farming practices that avoid the use of chemical fertilizers and pesticides. Therefore, the vitamins and all the macronutrients are organic molecules.) The transfer of carbon back to humans and other animals in the form of dietary molecules thus completes the carbon cycle. In this way, plants depend on humans and animals to provide CO_2 through the metabolism of nutrients, and animals depend on plants as the primary source of organic molecules needed for metabolism.

The cycling of **hydrogen** and **oxygen** atoms between plants and animals can also be traced (figure 3.1). Hydrogen and oxygen, in addition to carbon, are vital components of organic

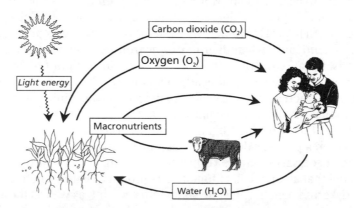

Figure 3.1 Nutrient recycling between plants and animals. Light energy from the sun is captured by plants in a process called photosynthesis, which combines carbon dioxide from the environment with water from the soil to make carbohydrates and other organic molecules. The sun's energy is retained within the chemical bonds that hold together the carbon, hydrogen, oxygen, and nitrogen atoms that comprise the macronutrients. A byproduct of photosynthesis is gaseous oxygen. After humans consume the macronutrients, they are broken down in the body to release the energy. The byproducts of nutrient metabolism are carbon dioxide and water, which are recycled back into the environment, making them available for photosynthesis and energy capture once again.

molecules made by plants, so their transfer to humans and other animals occurs when food is consumed. Oxygen (O_2) is also shuttled from plants to animals as gaseous oxygen in the atmosphere. Hydrogen is recycled back to plants primarily through uptake of water (H_2O) from the soil, while oxygen can return to plants as H_2O or as CO_2 from the atmosphere. The recycling of nutrients, therefore, is completely dependent on the ability of carbon, hydrogen, and oxygen atoms to combine and recombine into the various molecules that interact between plants and animals.

In addition to carbon, hydrogen, and oxygen, proteins and some vitamins contain **nitrogen** atoms, which are also recycled in the environment through pathways not shown in figure 3.1. Some plants are able to capture nitrogen gas from the atmosphere and incorporate it in their tissues. Nitrogen can also be taken up from the soil into the root system. Once inside the plant, nitrogen is incorporated into amino acids, vitamins, and other organic molecules, which are then consumed by humans and other animals. After the nitrogen-containing molecules are metabolized, nitrogen is recycled back into the environment by excretion in urine and feces.

Minerals are also essential nutrients that are recycled between plants and animals. Recall that the essential minerals are among the earthly elements and contain no carbon, hydrogen, oxygen, or nitrogen. Most minerals taken up by plants are present in the soil in which the plants are grown. Some minerals are abundant in the ocean and are transferred to humans through the consumption of marine plants and fish. The majority of minerals are recycled back into the environment by excretion in urine and feces, although some minerals exit the body through sweat and other bodily secretions.

Topic 3.3

Nutrients as Energy Distributors

> **Key Points**
>
> How is energy in food transformed into work in the body?
> What is ATP and why is it considered an "energy broker"?
> Can energy be stored in the body?

The inherent energy in carbohydrates, proteins, and triglycerides exists in the chemical bonds that hold together the carbon, hydrogen, oxygen, and nitrogen atoms that comprise each molecule. As carbohydrates are being assembled during photosynthesis, the atoms in CO_2 and H_2O are rearranged so that the sun's energy is captured within the chemical bonds. Further "processing" within the plant cells converts some of the carbohydrate into triglycerides and proteins. Triglycerides have the ability to store more energy in their chemical bonds than carbohydrates or proteins. Hence, triglycerides are considered **energy-dense** nutrients.

Once inside the body's cells, the molecular bonds are cleaved and the energy is released for the body to use. Figure 3.2 shows the major metabolic pathways involved in the release of energy from dietary carbohydrate, protein, and triglyceride. Notice that glucose, amino acids, and fatty acids are the primary components of the macronutrients and represent the chemical form of each nutrient that participates in energy metabolism. Written as a chemical formula, the complete breakdown of carbohydrate and subsequent release of its energy is the exact reverse of photosynthesis:

$$Carbohydrate + O_2 \rightarrow CO_2 + H_2O + Energy$$

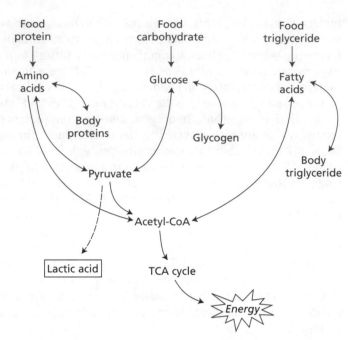

Figure 3.2 Macronutrient metabolism. After dietary protein, carbohydrate, and triglyceride are consumed, they are broken down to acetyl-CoA for entry into the tricarboxylic acid (TCA) cycle and the release of energy. Entry of dietary nutrients into the TCA cycle and complete oxidation to CO_2 and H_2O is called aerobic metabolism. Conversion of glucose to pyruvate is called glycolysis; further conversion to lactic acid occurs without oxygen and is called anaerobic metabolism. Under certain conditions, pyruvate may be converted to glucose in a process called gluconeogenesis. Macronutrients may be stored in the body as glycogen (in liver and muscle) and triglyceride (in adipose).

Because oxygen is required for this process to occur, the term **oxidation** is often used to describe the complete "burning" of carbohydrates, proteins, and triglycerides within the body's cells. Another term used to describe the oxidation of macronutrients to CO_2 and H_2O is **aerobic metabolism**.

During aerobic metabolism, each macronutrient is converted to a molecule called **acetyl–CoA**, which is then metabolized in a series of chemical reactions called the **tricarboxylic acid (TCA) cycle** (figure 3.2). The TCA cycle is also known as the citric acid cycle or Krebs' cycle, named after the biochemist who first described it in 1937. The central function of the TCA cycle is the complete oxidation of acetyl-CoA to CO_2 and H_2O. Although energy can be released from the macronutrients by other means, the TCA cycle accounts for about two-thirds of the energy captured from the diet and used in the body. Moreover, the TCA cycle is the only part of energy metabolism that requires oxygen.

The breakdown of glucose to pyruvate is called **glycolysis** and is an important step in energy metabolism because it does not require oxygen. A limited amount of energy is released in glycolysis, but much of the original energy remains in the chemical bonds of pyruvate. Only when enough oxygen is present in cells will pyruvate be converted to acetyl-CoA for entry into the TCA cycle. If oxygen is lacking, pyruvate is converted to **lactic acid** instead of acetyl-CoA, causing the build up of lactic acid in the cells (figure 3.2). The breakdown of glucose to lactic acid is called **anaerobic metabolism** because it occurs in the absence of oxygen. Anaerobic metabolism is an important pathway because it allows for energy to be released from macronutrients in cells that lack the TCA cycle (such as red blood cells) or in cells deprived of oxygen (such as tired muscle cells).

In a similar manner to glucose, some amino acids are converted to pyruvate prior to acetyl-CoA or lactic acid (figure 3.2). This is an important regulatory step because it allows glucose to be made from amino acids and vice versa (note the two-way arrows showing the bidirectional chemical reactions). Interconversion of glucose and amino acids provides cells with the opportunity to redistribute energy into forms that are needed at the moment. For example, it may be necessary to make glucose from amino acids when blood glucose levels drop too low between meals or during long-term fasting. The term **gluconeogenesis** is used to describe the conversion of pyruvate to glucose. Notice that dietary fatty acids cannot be converted to pyruvate and therefore cannot be made into glucose or amino acids. So the only possible fate of fatty acids is direct conversion to acetyl-CoA.

Despite the efficiency with which cells liberate energy from the macronutrients, the energy cannot be used directly in chemical reactions in the same way that light energy is directly used in photosynthesis. Instead, the energy released from acetyl-CoA is transferred to another molecule called **adenosine triphosphate** or ATP. The TCA cycle therefore "produces" ATP during the oxidation of acetyl-CoA. As with the dietary macronutrients, the energy is retained in the chemical bonds of ATP. But unlike the macronutrients, ATP can directly participate in the body's chemical reactions and, by doing so, provide the fuel that is required for body functions such as muscle movement, brain function, and many other vital functions. Thus, ATP can be thought of as an energy broker or distributor because of its pivotal role in receiving and transferring nutrient energy into usable cellular energy.

Although cells require a constant supply of energy for normal function, people do not eat continuously. Fortunately, some nutrients can be temporarily stored in the body to be used later when there is no incoming nutrients from the diet. Excess dietary carbohydrate can be converted to **glycogen** and stored in the liver and muscle, and excess dietary triglyceride can be stored in adipose (figure 3.2). While muscle protein can be broken down to amino acids and used for energy, this is not a primary function of muscle and is therefore not considered a primary storage form of dietary energy.

Application

The clinical symptoms that develop when energy metabolism malfunctions can often be used as a diagnostic tool. For example, when a person suffers a myocardial infarction (heart attack), the heart is unable to pump enough blood to deliver adequate amounts of oxygen to the tissues. Consequently, aerobic metabolism decreases and cells begin using anaerobic metabolism as a backup system for generating ATP for cell survival. The result is elevated concentrations of lactic acid in the blood, which can easily be diagnosed by measuring lactic acid in a blood sample. As one might predict, elevated blood lactic acid occurs in other disorders of the circulatory system, such as uncontrolled hemorrhage or pulmonary embolism, that diminish oxygen delivery to cells. Another example is a genetic condition that interferes with conversion of glucose to pyruvate during glycolysis. For most cells this is not a problem because fatty acids and amino acids can be used as energy sources in aerobic metabolism. However, red blood cells are unique because they can only use glucose for energy and are solely dependent on glycolysis and anaerobic metabolism for their energy. In this case, the red blood cells cannot get enough energy to maintain normal function and are easily destroyed. Not surprisingly, the main clinical symptom of this genetic condition is hemolytic anemia (destruction of red blood cells).

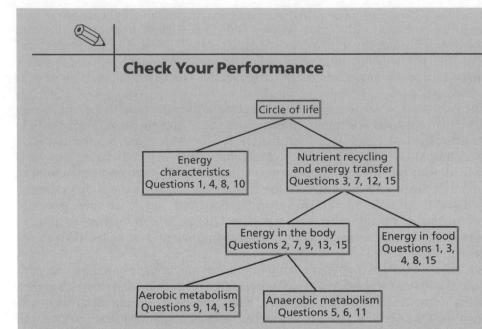

Check Your Performance

Chapter Test

True/False

1. Alcohol provides more energy per gram than carbohydrates
2. Carbohydrates can be directly stored in the body in adipose tissue
3. The term "organic" refers to molecules that contain nitrogen and are made only in plants
4. The standard unit of measurement for heat energy is the "calorie"
5. In general, lactic acid production increases when oxygen delivery to cells is limited

Multiple Choice

6. Anaerobic metabolism results in
   a. Pyruvate accumulation in cells
   b. The production of CO_2 and H_2O
   c. The release of energy from carbohydrate
   d. All of the above
7. Conversion of pyruvate to glucose is called
   a. Gluconeogenesis
   b. Glycopyrosis
   c. Glycolysis
   d. Pyrolysis
8. How much energy is in a large chocolate chip cookie containing 19 grams of carbohydrate, 1 gram of protein, and 5 grams of fat?
   a. 25 kilocalories
   b. 125 kilocalories
   c. 130 kilocalories
   d. 200 kilocalories

9. About two-thirds of all dietary energy is released in the body by
   a. The TCA cycle
   b. Photosynthesis
   c. Anaerobic metabolism
   d. Lactic acid production
10. Energy is broadly defined as
   a. The ability to give off heat
   b. The amount of light produced by the sun
   c. The amount of heat in 1 gram of water
   d. The ability to do work

Short Answer

11. Studies have shown that lactic acid can build up in muscles of sedentary people who suddenly engage in physical activity. What might be a likely explanation?
12. In nutrient recycling, how are hydrogen atoms shuttled between plants and animals?
13. With regard to cell metabolism, why is ATP considered an "energy broker"?
14. What is the tricarboxylic acid (TCA) cycle?

Essay

15. Describe how energy from the sun is used by humans to support life

Further Reading

Lehninger, A.I. (1971) *Bioenergetics*. W.A. Benjamin, Menlo Park, CA.

Mitchell, M.C. & Herlong, H.F. (1986) Alcohol and nutrition. *Annual Review of Nutrition*, 6, 457–74.

Nelson, D.L. & Cox, M.M. (2000) *Lehninger Principles of Biochemistry*, 3th ed. Worth Publishers, New York.

Nestle, M. (1997) Alcohol guidelines for chronic disease prevention: from prohibition to moderation. *Nutrition Today*, 32, 86–92.

Van der Meer, I.M., Bovy, A.G. & Bosch, D. (2001) Plant-based raw material: improved food quality for better nutrition via plant genomics. *Current Opinions in Biotechnology*, 12, 488–92.

Chapter 4

Nutrient Availability

Maintaining good health depends on a constant and adequate supply of nutrients. The availability of food is a critical factor contributing to the health of populations worldwide. It is estimated that nearly one billion people are undernourished because of the lack of food. Even in economically developed countries where the food supply is abundant, isolated pockets of malnutrition exist because access to food is limited. This chapter addresses the factors that contribute to food shortages and their impact on health. Also addressed in this chapter is how the governments of most developed countries strive to ensure adequate nutrient intake of their populations through nutrition education programs. The hallmark of these programs is the development of dietary recommendations designed for the general population. Nutrient availability can also be enhanced by consuming dietary supplements—isolated nutrients sold as powders or pills. While consuming whole foods is usually the most desirable way to obtain nutrients, taking a nutrient supplement may be warranted under certain conditions.

Essential Background

❖ Role of vitamins and minerals in supporting body functions (Chapter 1)
❖ Food sources of essential nutrients (Chapter 2)

Topic 4.1

Global Food Availability

Key Points

What causes food shortages worldwide?
What is famine?
What are the major effects of food shortages on human health?

At present, there is enough food produced in the world to adequately feed the entire earth's population, yet 55,000 people die of starvation each day. The problem is that the world's food supply is not equitably distributed. Therefore, some populations have more than enough food while others have too little. Although having too much food can be blamed for obesity and its health consequences, more people worldwide suffer from the ill effects of **food shortages**. Long-term or chronic food shortages are caused by overpopulation in certain regions of the world and lack of resources to support those populations. Food shortages can also be caused by more immediate events such as

Country	Males	Females
Japan	77.6	84.3
France	74.9	83.6
Australia	76.8	82.2
Spain	75.3	82.1
Canada	76.2	81.9
Netherlands	75.0	81.1
Singapore	75.1	80.8
Greece	75.5	80.5
Germany	73.7	80.1
Israel	76.2	79.9
UK	74.7	79.7
USA	73.8	79.7
Cuba	73.5	77.4
Mexico	71.0	77.1
Republic of Korea	69.2	76.3
Russian Federation	62.7	74.0
Romania	65.1	73.5
Saudi Arabia	71.0	72.6
Brazil	63.7	71.7
China	68.1	71.3
Indonesia	66.6	69.0
Egypt	64.2	65.8
India	59.6	61.2
Cambodia	52.2	55.4
South Africa	47.3	49.7
Ethiopia	41.4	43.1
Sierra Leone	33.2	35.4

Table 4.1 Life expectency (years) in selected countries, 1999

natural disasters, wars, and civil conflicts. Life expectancy in countries around the world (table 4.1) tends to reflect the distribution of food worldwide.

The human population is growing at a current rate of about 80 million individuals per year. About 1 billion people inhabited the earth in 1800, which increased to about 2 billion by 1900. There are now about 6 billion people living on the earth, and there appears to be no sign that the growth rate will slow in the near future. The vast majority of the growth is occurring in underdeveloped countries, where about three-quarters of the world's population currently live. The population growth is now occurring at a rate exceeding economic growth in many countries, resulting in increased poverty and a widening disparity between developed and underdeveloped countries. Most of the usable farmland worldwide is currently being used, and the growing population is causing farmland to be sacrificed for housing and industry. While it is currently possible for the global supply of food to provide adequate nutrients and total energy worldwide, unequal distribution of food is responsible for food shortages. Furthermore, some estimates show that food production has begun to lag behind population growth. The overall result is that overpopulation will continue to create food shortages in underdeveloped countries unless the growth rate slows down. Based on examples in many developing countries, most experts agree that the population growth rate will slow only when economic conditions improve and people have enough to eat.

Famine is a term given to widespread food shortages caused by natural disasters or human-induced events such as war or other social hardship. Food shortages that result from these events are almost always attributed to crop failure. The Irish potato famine of 1840–50 caused an

Table 4.2 Nutrient deficiency diseases commonly caused by food shortages

Deficiency disease	Key nutrient	Physiological effects
Ariboflavinosis	Riboflavin	Inflammation of eyes, lips, mouth, tongue Skin lesions Mental confusion
Beriberi	Thiamin	Nerve degeneration Cardiovascular alterations Poor muscle coordination
Goiter	Iodine	Enlarged thyroid gland Poor growth in children Mental retardation
Iron-deficiency anemia	Iron	Weakness and fatigue Poor growth in children Inability to maintain body temperature
Pellagra	Niacin	Dermatitis Diarrhea Dementia
Rickets (in children) Osteomalacia (in adults)	Vitamin D	Impaired bone formation in children resulting in bowed legs Weakened bones in adults
Scurvy	Vitamin C	Poor wound healing Bleeding gums Painful joints
Xerophthalmia	Vitamin A	Impaired vision and blindness Poor growth in children Dry skin

estimated 2 million deaths and forced nearly as many people to immigrate to other countries. Several million people have died in India during the last century because of famine caused by cyclones that frequently destroy India's crops. But the worst famine in human history occurred in China in 1958–61 when an estimated 30–40 million died as a result of failed social mandates and bizarre agricultural practices that dramatically reduced food production. Although these famine statistics are startling, they pale in comparison to the nearly 1 billion people worldwide who go to bed hungry each night because of chronic food shortages.

The impact of decreased food availability on human health depends on the extent and severity of nutrient deficiency. One of the most common deficiencies observed in developing countries is protein-energy malnutrition as described in Chapter 2. In addition, several other nutrient deficiency diseases are associated with food shortages and they are listed in table 4.2. While prolonged deficiency of many of these nutrients can eventually cause death, infections that accompany nutrition deficiencies often cause **diarrhea** and respiratory disease leading to death. Diarrhea alone is the primary cause of death of children in developing countries. It is also important to recognize that nutrient deficiencies can occur in developed countries despite an abundant food supply. Poverty and economic instability as well as disabilities and poor health can make it difficult for individuals to acquire and prepare food, thus leading to nutrient deficiencies. In the United States, several programs have been established to help make food more available to disadvantaged citizens, such as the Food Stamp Program, the National School Lunch Program, and the Special Supplemental Nutrition Program for Women, Infants, and Children (WIC).

Topic 4.2

Dietary Recommendations

Key Points

What is the purpose of creating dietary recommendations?
In what ways do dietary recommendations increase nutrient availability?
Why was the Food Guide Pyramid developed?

To maintain public health, government agencies in developed countries provide recommendations on what foods and how much people should eat. The concept of making dietary recommendations emerged from England in the mid 1800s when many people were moving into the cities to find work in the factories during the Industrial Revolution. The great influx of people created a situation similar to modern inner cities, with large numbers of homeless and undernourished people. The British government therefore established one of the first dietary recommendations in an attempt to keep their large industrial workforce healthy and productive. The United States government later applied a similar strategy for its military forces serving in the World War I. However, it was not until food shortages created by World War II that the United States issued the first dietary recommendations for its citizens in 1943. Today many countries have dietary recommendations tailored toward their own populations. And in the 1960s and 1970s, the World Health Organization and the Food and Agriculture Organization of the United Nations jointly issued dietary recommendations for worldwide use.

Dietary recommendations have generally been produced in two different forms—dietary standards and dietary guidelines. These terms have been used to distinguish their purpose and how recommendations are applied. **Dietary standards** represent the specific daily amount of essential nutrients that should be consumed to prevent deficiencies. They are based on both scientific research and expert opinion about how much of an essential nutrient is required by humans. However because each person's nutrient requirement is somewhat different, the dietary standards are set sufficiently high enough to apply to practically all healthy people within a group or population. Therefore, this approach means that dietary standards must exceed the minimum metabolic requirements of almost all individuals within the group or population for which they are intended. The dietary standards traditionally used in the United States are called the **Recommended Dietary Allowances** (RDAs) and were first published in 1943. Since the last edition of the RDAs in 1989, a large number of nutrition experts have argued that dietary standards should reflect not only the level of nutrients needed to prevent deficiencies, but also their contribution to reducing the risk of chronic diseases such as cancer and coronary heart disease. Consequently, a new set of dietary standards called the **Dietary Reference Intakes** (DRIs) have been developed in the United States that build on the RDA concept and are intended to replace the old RDAs.

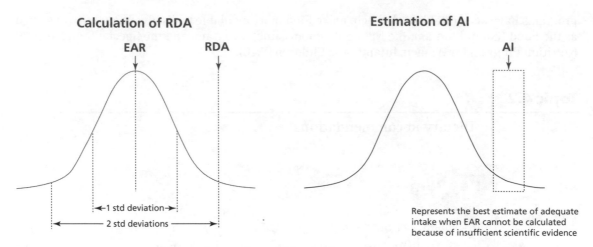

Figure 4.1 Determination of Dietary Reference Intake. The bell curve represents the normal distribution of intake for a nutrient in a population. When ample scientific evidence exists for the intake of a nutrient within a population or large group of people, the Recommended Dietary Allowance (RDA) is established (left panel). The RDA is set at 2 standard deviations above the Estimated Average Requirement (EAR). When the EAR cannot be determined because of insufficient data, Adequate Intake (AI) is used as the best estimate (right panel).

Establishing the DRIs for the essential nutrients is a systematic process based on scientific research, general observation, and expert opinion. The values currently used to represent the DRI for each essential nutrient are either the RDAs or Adequate Intake (AI). The ultimate goal is for every essential nutrient to have an RDA ascribed to it as the main "reference" value for the DRI. In cases where less information is known about a nutrient, an AI value is used until more research can be conducted and an RDA established with greater confidence. All DRI values, whether based on RDAs or AIs, have been separated by gender and life stage (age) to reflect differences in nutrient requirements. Very few scientific studies have been conducted to determine specific nutrient requirements in infants; therefore, AIs are used to represent DRIs for all of the essential nutrients for infants less than one year old. The current DRIs for the essential vitamins and minerals are presented in Appendix A.

RDAs are determined by first estimating the average nutrient requirement in a population or group of people (figure 4.1). This number is known as the Estimated Average Requirement (EAR). Obviously one cannot know for certain what this number would be unless the nutrient requirements for every person in the population was assessed, so information is generally collected from representative individuals within the larger population. Attempting to determine the EAR of a nutrient for an entire population or life-stage group is the single greatest difficulty in establishing the RDAs and is the reason why RDAs do not exist for all the essential nutrients. Assuming that an EAR has been determined with an acceptable level of confidence, the RDA for that nutrient is easily calculated as two standard deviations above the EAR. However, if insufficient evidence does not allow the EAR to be determined, the next best estimate is AI. The AIs are an approximation of the average nutrient intake that appears to be necessary for a population or group to maintain health (figure 4.1).

Another set of values, called the Tolerable Upper Intake Level (UL), are currently being developed to indicate the point at which a nutrient could be harmful. The UL for a nutrient is generally quite high and extremely difficult to reach by consuming food alone. However, the need for establishing ULs is necessary because of the growing use of vitamin and mineral supplements that

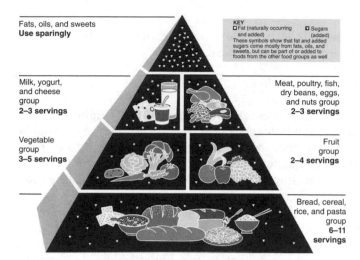

Figure 4.2 Food Guide Pyramid. Developed jointly by the United States Department of Agriculture and the Department of Health and Human Services, the Food Guide Pyramid provides recommendations on daily choices that, if followed, will meet all of the body's nutrient requirements for maintaining good health and reducing the risk of chronic disease. The Food Guide Pyramid is intended for use by the general public and does not require knowledge about the nutrient content of foods.

contain excessive amounts of essential nutrients. For example, the adult DRI for vitamin E is 15 mg/day, while the UL is 1,000 mg/day. Toxicity from vitamins and minerals can easily be avoided by consuming supplements only when necessary and by selecting supplements that do not exceed the DRI for any single nutrient.

Keep in mind that dietary standards were originally developed for use by health professionals in designing food strategies and diet plans for large groups of people and are not necessarily intended for use by consumers. Because most consumers have limited knowledge about nutrients, several food guides have been developed to help consumers make food choices that provide adequate nutrient intake. The most current food guide used in the United States is the **Food Guide Pyramid,** first published in 1992 (figure 4.2). The Food Guide Pyramid divides foods into groups based on their most abundant nutrients and physical characteristics. In addition, the Food Guide Pyramid provides a recommended number of servings from each food group needed each day for a healthy diet.

In contrast to dietary standards, **dietary guidelines** are more general in nature and are meant to reduce the risk of chronic diseases and to promote an individual's overall health and well being. Dietary guidelines represent advice for the public that is based on both scientific evidence and social concerns. Since 1980, the US Department of Agriculture and the Department of Health and Human Services have jointly published the **Dietary Guidelines for Americans.** Every five years the Dietary Guidelines are updated and the most recent edition was published in 2000. The Dietary Guidelines provide the basis for Federal nutrition policy and nutrition education activities. Specifically, the Guidelines provide advice for healthy Americans ages two years and over about food choices that promote health and reduce the risk of disease:

Aim for fitness
- Aim for a healthy weight
- Be physically active each day

Build a healthy base
- Let the Pyramid guide your food choices
- Choose a variety of grains daily, especially whole grains
- Choose a variety of fruits and vegetables daily
- Keep food safe to eat

Choose sensibly
- Choose a diet that is low in saturated fat and cholesterol and moderate in total fat
- Choose beverages and foods to moderate your intake of sugars
- Choose and prepare foods with less salt
- If you drink alcoholic beverages, do so in moderation

Another important set of guidelines in the United States is **Healthy People 2010**. Originally developed in 1990 by the US Department of Health and Human Services through an alliance with public and private health organizations, the primary goals of Healthy People 2010 are (i) to increase quality and years of healthy life and (ii) to eliminate health disparities. The goals are to be met through broad-based programs that promote healthy behaviors, encourage safe and healthy communities, assure access to quality health care, and reduce or prevent diseases.

Several other health organizations in the United States, such as the American Heart Association and the National Cancer Institute, have published their own dietary guidelines. Although all the dietary guidelines tend to make the same general recommendations, differences among them usually focus on nutrients most relevant to the organizations' causes. For example, the American Heart Association guidelines recommend limiting cholesterol intake, whereas the National Cancer Institute guidelines emphasize a diet high in fruits, vegetables, and fiber.

Topic 4.3 |

Dietary Supplements

Key Points

What are the different types of dietary supplements?
Are dietary supplements necessary for good health?
Are dietary supplements safe and reliable?

People consume dietary supplements for a variety of reasons. Many people take supplements because of ill health or to prevent nutrient deficiencies, while others take supplements with the belief that they somehow improve metabolic function or simply make them feel better. Whatever the reason, our desire for dietary supplements has created a multi-billion dollar industry in the United States. Despite such widespread popularity, few people realize that the manufacture and sale of supplements is largely unregulated, and little is known about their safety and effectiveness. The only requirements—set forth by the Dietary Supplement Health and Education Act of 1994—are that supplement packages include the words "dietary supplement" and that the label indicates the recommended serving size and the name and amount of each ingredient per serving. Other than these labeling requirements, there is no law that regulates what ingredients are used in dietary supplements. Many supplements are marketed as being "all natural," leading consumers to believe they are safe. However, dozens of deaths have occurred in recent years because of consumers' lack of understanding of what dietary supplements contain, their effect on metabolism, and their potential danger. Not all dietary supplements are inherently dangerous, and there are situations where taking a specific supplement may be warranted. However, the loose government regulations have allowed the marketplace to be flooded with products for which we have little or no information regarding their reliability and safety. The following discussion will focus on four major groups of dietary supplements: vitamins and minerals, proteins and amino acids, herbs and botanicals, and metabolic chemicals.

Because of the body's requirement for essential micronutrients, it may be necessary to include a **vitamin and mineral supplement** under certain conditions. Nutrition experts like to believe that all essential nutrients can be obtained from a well-balanced diet, but there are clearly situations when the body's micronutrient requirement is greater than that the diet can provide. An obvious example is the loss of blood during menstruation, which increases a woman's need for dietary iron to levels that are often difficult to achieve through food alone. Other examples include people who voluntarily restrict certain foods, such as vegetarians or habitual dieters. Whether nutrient limitations are due to metabolic reasons or dietary restriction, it is always best to know what specific nutrients are affected so that an appropriate supplement may be chosen. Strict vegetarians exclude animal products from their diet, so a supplement containing micronutrients found primarily in animal foods (such as vitamin B_{12}, vitamin D, iron, and zinc) may be warranted—a supplement containing vitamin C, on the other hand, would most likely be unnecessary. Taking vitamin and mineral supplements on a routine basis and without a valid reason can shift attention away from the importance of whole foods and create a false sense of security about health. Moreover, some vitamins and minerals can become toxic if consumed in excess. Such high levels are most often due to the inappropriate use of dietary supplements and are nearly impossible to achieve through consumption of whole foods.

Protein and **amino acid supplements** are popular among physically active people because of their promise to build muscle and improve performance. Unfortunately, this notion is one of the biggest misconceptions in nutrition. The only way to build muscle is to use muscle—taking a protein or amino acid supplement will not force muscle to grow or become stronger. This misconception is analogous to installing a larger gas tank on your car hoping it will increase its speed. Providing more gasoline will not increase your car's performance—only adjustments to the engine will do that. While physical activity does increase protein needs, these requirements are easily met from the protein found in a balanced diet. Protein intake for the average adult in the United States is already twice the requirement, so consuming expensive protein or amino acid supplements is quite unnecessary. High-protein diets also increase fluid needs and the risk of dehydration. Furthermore, some amino acid supplements have caused death from toxic levels of isolated amino acids and because of impurities in the amino acid preparations.

Herbs and other **botanical substances** have long been known to affect the body's metabolism. Ancient cultures used herbs as medicines, and many modern drugs are based on chemicals extracted from plants. Native Americans often treated pain by chewing on willow bark, which we now know contains the chemical acetylsalicylic acid—aspirin. The effect that plant substances have on the human body can be traced to specific chemicals. In this way, ingesting supplements made from plant materials is akin to taking drugs. When a patient is prescribed a drug, information has been collected and carefully evaluated regarding the drug's dose, its purity, and its specific effect on the body (including potential side effects). No such procedure exists in the manufacture and use of plant-derived supplements.

With the increasing popularity of alternative medicines in Western societies, many people are choosing to manage their own health and to treat their ailments with herbal remedies. For this approach to be successful, one must have knowledge about the risks and benefits of the chemicals in herbs and other botanical substances. The proper use of herbs, when administered by a skilled practitioner, can be effective in promoting good health. However, self-medication with herbs can be a dangerous and even deadly practice. The main problem is that the quality of herbs available to consumers is unknown—they have not been screened for authenticity or purity. It is clearly a "buyer beware" market for herbs. Furthermore, only a few herbs have been systematically studied for their effect on human metabolism, and their interactions with modern drugs and other supplements can enhance their harmful effects. Table 4.3 lists several herbs that have been used for medicinal

Table 4.3 Herbs and botanicals used for medicinal purposes[a]

Alfalfa ☠	Fenugreek	Pennyroyal ☠
Aloe	Feverfew	Peppermint
Arnica ☠	Fo-ti (he-shou-wu)	Red clover
Asafetida	Garlic ☺	Red raspberry
Astragalus	Gentian	Rose hips
Barberry	Ginger	Rutin
Bee pollen	Gingko biloba	Sarsaparilla
Black cohosh	Ginseng	Sassafras ☠
Black walnut	Goldenseal	Saw palmetto
Black pepper	Gotu kola	Scullcap ☠
Bladderwrack	Guarana	Senna
Borage ☠	Hawthorn berry ☠	Slippery elm
Burdock root ☠	Herbal teas ☠	Spirulina (blue green algae)
Caraway seed	Hops	Sumac ☠
Cascara sagrada	Horehound	Tea tree oil
Catnip	Hyssop	Turmeric
Cayenne	Jin bu huan ☠	Uva ursi ☠ (bear berry)
Chamomile	Juniper berry ☠	Valerian root
Chaparral ☠	Kelp ☠	White oak bark
Chickweed	Licorice ☠	White willow ☠
Comfrey root ☠	Lobelia ☠	Wood betony
Damiana ☠	Ma huang ☠	Yarrow
Dandelion	Marshmallow root	Yellow dock
Dong quai	Milk thistle	Yerbemate
Echinacea ☺	Mullein	Yohimbe ☠
Evening primrose oil	Nettle	
Eyebright	Parsley	
Fennel	Pau d'arco ☠ (ipe roxo, lapacho, taheebo tea)	

[a] No known toxicity is indicated by ☺; proven toxicity is indicated by ☠.

purposes. Note that the only two herbs having no known side effects with prolonged use are echinacea and garlic. Perhaps a risk/benefit analysis can help determine whether you should take an herbal supplement and which ones are most appropriate for your ailment. You should use as much care and apply the same level of scrutiny in choosing herbal supplements as you do in choosing the foods you eat.

Several **metabolic chemicals** found in the body are manufactured and sold as dietary supplements. These substances are not essential nutrients and their absence from the diet does not produce deficiency symptoms. Some people take these supplements with the belief that the body does not make enough for optimal health or that providing excess will increase the body's performance. Some of these metabolic chemicals include carnitine, coenzyme Q_{10}, DHEA, inositol, lipoic acid, and melatonin. Each of these substances performs a specific function in the body, so having knowledge about their function is critical in selecting the most appropriate supplement for the condition you wish to treat. For example, glucosamine sulfate and chondroitin sulfate are normally found in the cartilage of joints. Many people believe that taking these chemicals as supplements relieves arthritis pain and increases flexibility and movement. Unlike herbal supplements which contain chemicals foreign to the body, metabolic chemicals taken in moderate amounts are unlikely to be harmful. Nevertheless, the same level of caution should be used when purchasing these supplements to assess their purity and quality.

Application

Many types of clinical situations prevent patients from eating or digesting food. In these cases, nutrients must be made available by alternative methods in order to meet the body's basic needs. **Parenteral feeding** refers to the method of introducing nutrients intravenously. This delivery system bypasses the gastrointestinal tract and provides nutrients directly into the bloodstream. Parenteral feeding is best for patients suffering from intestinal disorders, those that cannot ingest food, severe burns patients, and underweight premature infants. Several nutrient solutions are commercially available, each having a different mixture of nutrients designed for specific clinical conditions. Complications do arise from parenteral feeding, such as nutrient deficiencies, fluid imbalances, liver dysfunction, gallstones, and decreased bone mass, although some of the causes are not completely known. Many of the complications can be avoided or minimized with proper care and experience of the health care provider. Another alternative feeding method is **enteral feeding**, in which nutrient mixtures are delivered into the gastrointestinal tract by way of a tube introduced through the nasal passages or placed surgically into the stomach or small intestine. The greatest advantage of enteral feeding is that the structure and function of the gastrointestinal tract is largely preserved. Nutrient solutions are commercially available, although homogenized whole foods can also be used. Most of the complications arising from enteral feeding tend to be less severe than parenteral feeding and include nausea, vomiting, diarrhea, and constipation.

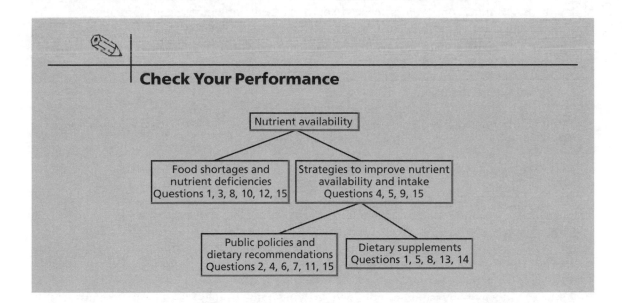

Check Your Performance

Nutrient availability

Food shortages and nutrient deficiencies
Questions 1, 3, 8, 10, 12, 15

Strategies to improve nutrient availability and intake
Questions 4, 5, 9, 15

Public policies and dietary recommendations
Questions 2, 4, 6, 7, 11, 15

Dietary supplements
Questions 1, 5, 8, 13, 14

Chapter Test

True/False

1. Iron-deficiency anemia is a common problem associated with food shortages worldwide

2. The United States is the only economically developed country that provides dietary recommendations to its citizens

3. Famine is a term used to describe short-term food shortages caused by natural disasters such as floods or earthquakes

4. There is currently no set of dietary recommendations that are applied worldwide

5. All dietary supplements contain unknown chemicals and should never need to be taken

Multiple Choice

6. The Dietary Reference Intakes (DRIs)
   a. Have been used since 1943
   b. Are intended to replace the Food Guide Pyramid
   c. Apply to practically all healthy people
   d. All of the above

7. All of the following programs have been established in the United States to help ensure adequate nutrient availability <u>except</u>
   a. The Food Stamp Program
   b. The National School Lunch Program
   c. The Special Supplemental Nutrition Program for Women, Infants, and Children
   d. The Alcohol and Tobacco Voucher Program for Senior Citizens

8. Dietary supplements are best described as
   a. Isolated nutrients or other substances consumed in addition to a whole food diet
   b. Pills, liquids, or powders needed to optimize health and increase performance
   c. Concentrated natural substances needed for increased energy and mental function
   d. Plant-derived substances required for chronic disease prevention

9. "Parenteral feeding" refers to
   a. Infant feeding techniques
   b. Intravenous nutrient delivery
   c. Delivery of nutrients through a stomach tube
   d. Caring for elderly parents

10. The primary cause of death among children worldwide is
   a. Diabetes
   b. Hypertension
   c. Diarrhea
   d. Cancer

Short Answer

11. What are the three major recommendations outlined in the Dietary Guidelines for Americans?

12. What are some of the major causes of food shortages?

13. Explain why the vast majority of people living in the United States (including athletes) do not need to take protein supplements

14. What is the primary advantage of enteral feeding compared to parenteral feeding?

Essay

15. What is the difference between dietary standards and dietary guidelines?

Further Reading

American Dietetic Association (2001) Position of the American Dietetic Association: food fortification and dietary supplements. *Journal of the American Dietetic Association*, 101, 115–25.

Dietary Guidelines for Americans (2000) US Department of Agriculture and Health and Human Services. (http://www.nal.usda.gov/fnic/dga/index.html) Accessed 26 Jan 2002.

Freeland-Graves, J. & Nitzke, S. (2002) Position of the American Dietetic Association: total diet approach to communicating food and nutrition information. *Journal of the American Dietetic Association*, 102, 100–8.

Fuhrman, M.P., Winkler, M. & Biesemeier, C. (2001) The American Society for Parenteral and Enteral Nutrition (ASPEN) standards of practice for nutrition support dietitians. *Journal of the American Dietetic Association*, 101, 825–32.

Greene, H.L., Prior, T. & Frier, H.I. (2001) Foods, health claims, and the law: comparison of the United States and Europe. *Obesity Research*, 9(Suppl. 4), 276S–83S.

Hathcock, J. (2001) Dietary supplements: how they are used and regulated. *Journal of Nutrition*, 131, 1114S–17S.

Healthy People 2010. Office of Disease Prevention and Health Promotion, US Department of Health and Human Services. (http://www.health.gov/healthypeople) Accessed 31 Jan 2002.

Koffman, D.M., Bazzarre, T., Mosca, L., Redberg, R., Schmid, T. & Wattigney, W.A. (2001) An evaluation of Choose to Move 1999: an American Heart Association physical activity program for women. *Archives of Internal Medicine*, 161, 2193–9.

Krauss, R.M., Eckel, R.H., Howard, B., *et al.* (2000) AHA Dietary Guidelines: revision 2000. A statement for healthcare professionals from the Nutrition Committee of the American Heart Association. *Circulation*, 102, 2284–99.

Massey, P.B. (2002) Dietary supplements. *Medical Clinics of North America*, 86, 127–47.

Radimer, K.L., Subar, A.F. & Thompson F.E. (2000) Nonvitamin, nonmineral dietary supplements: issues and findings from NHANES III. *Journal of the American Dietetic Association*, 100, 447–54.

Part II

Nutrients in the Body

Chapter 5

Nutrient Capture and Assimilation

All living things must eat in order to survive. The simple act of eating, however, is only the first step in which humans and other animals capture nutrients from the environment. Once inside the body, foods are broken down so that nutrients contained in food can be made available for absorption into the body's cells. The mechanical and chemical processes that break down food and convert its nutrients to absorbable forms are collectively known as **digestion**.

Essential Background

❖ Nutrients and their functions (Chapter 1)
❖ Major forms of nutrients in food (Chapters 1 and 2)
❖ The blood and lymphatic circulatory systems
❖ Transfer of energy from the environment to the body (Chapters 2 and 3)

Topic 5.1

Digestion

> ### Key Points
>
> What is the gastrointestinal tract and how is it organized?
> What is the primary purpose of digestion?
> How do enzymes, saliva, and bile function in digestion?
> What are the nutrient products of digestion?

Digestion of food occurs within the **gastrointestinal (GI) tract**, also known as the intestinal tract, digestive tract, gut, and alimentary canal. It is essentially a tube about 9 meters (30 feet) long that is open to the environment. The cells that line the GI tract are actually epithelial cells, the same type of cells that make up skin and cover the outside of our bodies. When food is consumed, it is still technically outside the body until the digested products are absorbed into the body's cells. As discussed earlier, some food components such as dietary fiber are not absorbed and merely ride through the GI tract. The organs—or sections—of the GI tract are the mouth, esophagus, stomach, small intestine, large intestine, rectum, and anus (figure 5.1). Ringlike muscles called **sphincters** are located between sections in the GI tract and help to regulate the flow of food. In addition to the main digestive tube, additional organs participate in digestion and are considered part of the GI

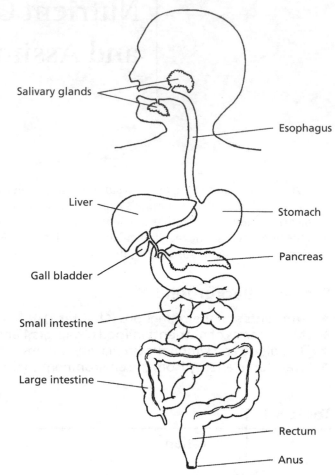

Salivary glands

Esophagus

Liver

Stomach

Pancreas

Gall bladder

Small intestine

Large intestine

Rectum

Anus

Figure 5.1   The gastrointestinal tract. Divided into sections, the gastrointestinal tract is essentially a long tube in which food is digested and nutrients absorbed into the body. Following the mouth is the esophagus, stomach, small intestine, large intestine, rectum, and anus. The salivary glands, liver, gallbladder, and pancreas are accessory organs that produce and release digestive juices into the gastrointestinal tract.

tract. These **accessory organs** are the salivary glands, liver, gallbladder, and pancreas. The salivary glands are located in the mouth, whereas the liver, gallbladder, and pancreas are connected to the small intestine. The accessory organs are necessary because they produce digestive juices that are released into the GI tract when foods are consumed.

Digestion begins in the mouth when food is chewed and broken into smaller pieces—a process called **mastication**. Saliva is released by the salivary glands and contains two enzymes, **salivary amylase** and **lingual lipase**, which begin the chemical breakdown of starch and triglyceride, respectively (figure 5.2). The simple chemical definition of enzymes is proteins that speed up and regulate chemical reactions in the body. Salivary amylase and lingual lipase are only partially effective at digesting starch and triglyceride because they are neutralized by stomach acid. Another function of saliva is to provide lubrication to low-moisture foods. After food is swallowed, it enters the esophagus and is propelled down by a series of wavelike, rhythmic muscular contractions called **peristalsis**.

Separating the esophagus and stomach is the gastroesophageal sphincter. It relaxes to allow food to enter the stomach, then closes to prevent the backflow of food into the esophagus. The stomach is a muscular pouch that acts as a mixing chamber for food, saliva, and digestive juices

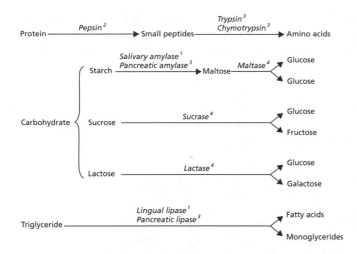

Figure 5.2 Enzymatic digestion of nutrients. The final (absorbable) products of digestion are amino acids, monosaccharides, fatty acids, and monoglycerides. Superscripts indicate the tissues in which the enzymes are produced: [1]salivary glands; [2]stomach; [3]pancreas; [4]small intestine.

made in the stomach. The semiliquid food mass formed during mixing in the stomach is called **chyme**. The gastric secretions made by the stomach include **hydrochloric acid** and the enzyme **pepsin**. Hydrochloric acid and pepsin work together to break down proteins into smaller **peptides** (figure 5.2). The stomach itself is mostly protein, but it is protected from self-digestion by a thick layer of mucus. Occasionally the gastroesophageal sphincter does not close properly and stomach acid can reflux back into the esophagus causing "heartburn."

The release of chyme into the small intestine occurs very slowly and is regulated by the pyloric sphincter. The small intestine is about 6 meters (20 feet), the longest section of the GI tract. The inner wall of the small intestine is covered with fingerlike projections called **villi**, which in turn are covered with **microvilli**. Consequently, the surface area of the small intestine is greatly increased to help facilitate nutrient absorption. It has been calculated that the total surface area of the small intestine is about 300 m^2—the size of a tennis court! Most nutrients are absorbed in the small intestine. Because of the brushlike appearance of microvilli when viewed under the microscope, the inner wall of the small intestine is often referred to as the brush border.

As the acidic chyme enters the small intestine, it is neutralized by **bicarbonate** produced in the pancreas and secreted into the small intestine. Digestive juices from the pancreas also contain enzymes that continue the breakdown of protein, starch, and triglyceride (figure 5.2). **Trypsin** and **chymotrypsin** further cleave small peptides into amino acids. **Pancreatic amylase** continues the job started by the salivary amylase by converting starch into maltose. Epithelial cells of the brush border make the enzymes **maltase**, **sucrase**, and **lactase**, which break down the disaccharides maltose, sucrose, and lactose, respectively. To help facilitate the action of pancreatic lipase, the liver makes a "detergent" called **bile**, which helps to break lipid droplets into smaller particles. Bile is stored in the gallbladder and is released into the small intestine when dietary lipids are present. Thus, the final breakdown products of digestion—those nutrients that can be absorbed—are amino acids, monosaccharides, fatty acids, and monoglycerides. Vitamins and minerals present in food do not require further breakdown and are absorbed intact.

Any undigested food remnants travel to the large intestine through the ileocecal sphincter. **Bacteria**—or microflora—that normally live in the large intestine have the ability to use the "left-overs" as fuel, often producing gas as a byproduct. Feces are formed in the large intestine from food residue, bacteria, and dead cells that slough off during passage of food. The large intestine is also the site of water absorption. **Dietary fiber** can help attract and retain water in the large intestine, making the feces soft and easier to eliminate. Inadequate fiber or fluids in the diet can produce dry, hard feces and are the primary causes of constipation. The feces eventually travel to the rectum where they are stored until being released from the body by voluntary control of the anal sphincter.

Topic 5.2

Mechanisms of Nutrient Absorption

> **Key Points**
>
> What is passive diffusion, facilitated diffusion, and active transport?
> How does the absorption of water-soluble and fat-soluble nutrients differ?
> How do micelles help in lipid absorption?

Absorption refers to the movement of nutrients from the interior—or lumen—of the GI tract into the cells that line the surface of the small intestine. Some nutrients are completely absorbed under most conditions, whereas the absorption of other nutrients can be highly variable depending on intestinal contents and the interaction of nutrients. **Bioavailability** is a general term describing how well a nutrient is absorbed. The passage of water-soluble nutrients through the cell membrane can occur by three mechanisms: passive diffusion, facilitated diffusion, or active transport (figure 5.3).

   Passive diffusion occurs when the concentration of a nutrient is greater in the intestinal lumen than inside the cell. Following a meal, the concentration of nutrients is usually higher in the intestinal lumen, causing some nutrients to move freely into the cell. The bioavailability of nutrients absorbed solely by passive diffusion will always be less than 100% because an equilibrium is eventually reached between the nutrient inside the cell and that remaining in the lumen. **Facilitated diffusion** is similar to passive diffusion, except that specific carrier proteins are needed

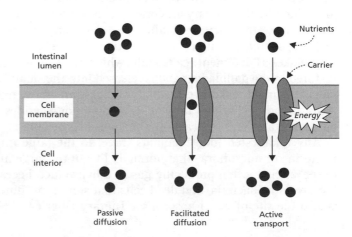

Figure 5.3 Mechanisms of nutrient absorption. Nutrients enter the intestinal cell by moving across the membrane from the intestinal lumen. Passive diffusion does not require a carrier protein or the input of energy. Facilitated diffusion requires a carrier protein but no input of energy. Active transport requires a carrier protein and the input of energy.

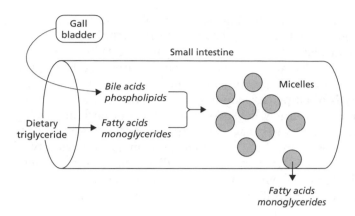

Figure 5.4   Micelle formation. The products of triglyceride digestion—fatty acids and monoglycerides—combine with bile acids and phospholipids from the gallbladder to form micelles. The tiny micelles act to "dissolve" the lipid so that it may enter the intestinal cell by passive diffusion.

to move some nutrients across the cell membrane. **Active transport** requires both a specific carrier protein and the input of energy. The advantage of active transport is that some nutrients are "pumped" into cells even when their concentration becomes greater inside the cell than in the intestinal lumen. Consequently, active transport can result in complete absorption of some nutrients.

Each water-soluble nutrient exhibits its own absorption characteristics. The amino acids are absorbed by either active transport or facilitated diffusion, whereas the water-soluble vitamins can be absorbed by all three mechanisms. Although mineral absorption is not well understood, all three mechanisms of absorption appear to occur among the minerals. Glucose and galactose are absorbed by active transport, whereas fructose is apparently absorbed by facilitated diffusion.

In contrast to water-soluble nutrients, fat-soluble nutrients require an additional step prior to absorption. The products of triglyceride digestion—fatty acids and monoglycerides—are first formed into tiny lipid droplets called **micelles** before they are absorbed by passive diffusion. Micelles are formed when fatty acids and monoglycerides from the diet combine with **bile** from the gallbladder. Bile contains a mixture of **bile acids** (made in the liver from cholesterol) and **phospholipids** that help "dissolve" the dietary lipid (figure 5.4). The bile acids and phospholipids act as detergents in a manner similar to washing greasy dishes with commercial detergents. The formation of micelles is necessary to break the dietary lipids into very small particles to allow absorption within the aqueous environment of the small intestine. Once inside the intestinal cell, the fatty acids and monoglycerides are reassembled into triglycerides. Dietary cholesterol and the fat-soluble vitamins also depend on micelle formation for absorption into the intestinal cell.

Problems with lipid absorption can occur when bile production and secretion are impaired. Normally the components of bile exist together in proportions that maximize fat solubility when released into the small intestine. However, when the balance is upset, the cholesterol becomes supersaturated, forming microscopic crystals that eventually develop into gall "stones." Gallstones can be too small to be seen with the naked eye (forming bile "sludge"), or they can be as large as golf balls. The gallbladder may contain a single stone or several hundred of various sizes. The formation of gallstones (cholelithiasis) is one of the most common pathological conditions affecting the digestive tract. Approximately 25 million Americans have confirmed gallstones, while many more people probably have them but experience no unpleasant symptoms and are unaware of them. This condition results in at least 400,000 gallbladder operations each year in the United States. Most gallstones are asymptomatic—they cause no pain and are considered "silent" stones. Gallstones are a problem only if they block the cystic duct or common bile duct that channel bile from the gallbladder to the small intestine. The obstruction causes pain (gallbladder colic) and can lead to inflammation (cholecystitis) and infection (cholangitis) of the gallbladder. The primary symptoms include abdominal pain, fever, and jaundice. Other symptoms can include fatty stools (because of poor fat absorption), bloating, nausea, vomiting, heartburn, and flatulence. When symptoms of gallstones are present, the primary treatment is surgical removal of the gallbladder. The surgery is often performed on an outpatient basis and patients usually return to their normal routines within a few days. Another treatment currently being explored is breaking up the gallstones by ultrasound shock waves. However, this treatment does not prevent the return of gallstones, whereas removal of the gallbladder eliminates the ability of stones to form. Some individuals without gallbladders may need to modify their diets to compensate, although most people suffer no ill effects of having no gallbladder. In fact, several mammal species do not have gallbladders, so bile flow occurs directly from the liver to the small intestine without being stored.

Topic 5.3

Nutrient Destinations

> **Key Points**
>
> How does the transport of water-soluble and fat-soluble nutrients differ?
> What tissues receive dietary amino acids, glucose, and triglyceride after absorption?
> What are chylomicrons?

Every cell in the body requires the influx of nutrients to maintain normal function. As nutrients are absorbed from the diet, they travel to the tissues where they are immediately used or stored for later use. Some nutrients that are stored in one tissue (such as glucose in the liver) may be released into the blood at a later time for use by another tissue (such as the brain). Indeed, a great network of "communication" exists among all tissues of the body. Integration of metabolism is a critical concept in understanding nutrition and will be discussed in the next two chapters. The current section will focus on how dietary nutrients enter the blood and are subsequently transported to tissues.

After absorption into the intestinal cell, water-soluble nutrients enter blood capillaries that converge into the **hepatic portal vein**. Connected to the hepatic portal vein is the **liver**, the first organ to receive water-soluble nutrients after absorption. Some nutrients are retained by the liver, while others pass through the liver and continue on in the **general circulation** for delivery to other tissues. Water-soluble vitamins and minerals, for example, quickly distribute among the body's tissues in response to the cellular requirements. Water-soluble vitamins and minerals are not stored in the body for very long, so those not immediately used are excreted in the urine. This phenomenon illustrates the importance of consistently consuming a well-balanced diet that contains a variety of vitamins and minerals.

Dietary amino acids are also transported directly to the liver after absorption (figure 5.5). Amino acids not immediately used by the liver are sent into the general circulation and transported to

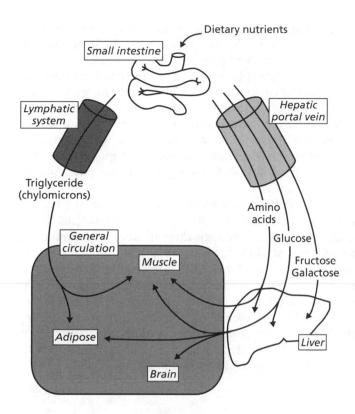

Figure 5.5 Nutrient transport. After absorption, amino acids and monosaccharides are transported directly to the liver via the hepatic portal vein. The liver retains some glucose and amino acids, while the remainder enters the general circulation for delivery to other tissues. Absorbed triglyceride is packaged as chylomicrons and transported first in the lymphatic system before entering the general circulation for delivery to the body's tissues.

other tissues for protein synthesis. Excess amino acids are transported in the blood back to the liver where they are broken down and used for energy. In the usual American diet, the majority of amino acids are used for protein synthesis rather than energy.

About two-thirds of dietary glucose is retained by the liver when first absorbed (figure 5.5). The other one-third passes through the liver and can be taken up by virtually all tissues of the body, although the **brain, muscle,** and, to a lesser extent, **adipose** are the biggest users of circulating glucose. The other dietary monosaccharides—fructose and galactose—are mostly captured by the liver and metabolized. Consequently, the concentration of fructose and galactose in circulating blood is normally quite low. The rapid metabolism of fructose and galactose by the liver ensures that essentially all digestible carbohydrate will be utilized most efficiently and that only glucose contributes to "blood sugar."

Unlike water-soluble nutrients, the fat-soluble nutrients cannot directly enter the aqueous bloodstream. They must first associate with specialized proteins within the intestinal cell to form lipoprotein complexes called **chylomicrons.** This lipid–protein association allows fat-soluble nutrients to become, in a sense, "water-soluble" for transport within the aqueous environment of the body. The chylomicrons first enter the lymph ducts connected to the intestinal cells and travel via the **lymphatic system** to the left subclavian vein near the heart (figure 5.5). At this point the chylomicrons enter the bloodstream for transport and delivery of the fat-soluble nutrients throughout the body. Because triglyceride is the most abundant dietary lipid, chylomicrons are composed primarily of triglyceride. But they are also the main transport vehicle for dietary cholesterol and fat-soluble vitamins.

The absorption and transport of dietary triglyceride in the form of chylomicrons is a highly efficient way of capturing and storing energy from the diet. Unlike the majority of water-soluble nutrients, which go directly to the liver for "processing," chylomicrons bypass the liver and thus have the opportunity to deliver dietary triglyceride in unaltered form to adipose, muscle, and other tissues. From an evolutionary point of view, transporting this energy-dense nutrient from the small intestine directly to peripheral tissues is energy efficient and highly advantageous for survival of a species. For example, generations ago when humans gathered their own food, it was much more difficult to meet nutrient needs during the winter months when food was scarce. Being able to directly transport dietary triglyceride to adipose tissue for storage during the warmer months ensured enough reserve energy when nutrient intake was limited. However, in modern societies where the food supply is accessible and abundant, this process is perhaps too efficient and promotes the storage of excess energy in adipose tissue.

In addition to chylomicrons, three other classes of lipoproteins exist in human blood: very low density lipoproteins (VLDL), low density lipoproteins (LDL), and high density lipoproteins (HDL). Each class of lipoprotein performs a different function, although they all have in common the ability to transport lipid in the aqueous environment of the bloodstream. The different classes of lipoproteins contain varying proportions of lipids and proteins. VLDL are smaller then chylomicrons and function to deliver triglyceride made in the liver to other tissues. Smaller still are LDL, which contain mostly cholesterol. LDL are actually remnants of VLDL when the VLDL become depleted of triglyceride after delivery to tissues. LDL are considered the "bad cholesterol" among health care professionals because of their high cholesterol content. Strategies to lower blood cholesterol are aimed specifically at lowering LDL. Finally, the smallest lipoproteins are HDL, which function to pick up excess cholesterol from peripheral tissues and transport it back to the liver where it can be excreted from the body.

Application

Lactose intolerance is a condition in which individuals are unable to digest lactose, the primary sugar in milk and dairy products. This inability is due to a deficiency of the enzyme lactase in the small intestine. Infants generally have adequate amounts of lactase, although enzyme production tends to decrease as people get older. Symptoms of lactose intolerance—including nausea, cramps, bloating, gas, and diarrhea—usually begin a few minutes after consuming foods or beverages containing lactose. The severity of the symptoms depends on how much lactose is consumed and the extent of lactase deficiency. Complete avoidance of milk and dairy products can minimize symptoms, but also limits food choices rich in calcium and may not be entirely necessary. The chemical processes used in making cheese and yogurt, for example, remove most of the lactose present in milk. Lactose-intolerant individuals should also be aware of nondairy foods high in calcium, such as shrimp, oysters, sardines, molasses, broccoli, and certain other green leafy vegetables. An alternative approach is to purchase the lactase enzyme in liquid or tablet form. The lactase liquid can be added to milk prior to drinking, whereas lactase tablets can be ingested with food at mealtime.

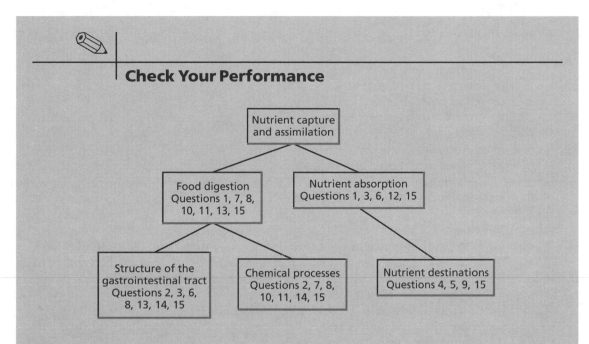

Check Your Performance

Chapter Test

True/False

1. Micelles are formed in the small intestine in response to a high-protein meal

2. Bacterial growth in the large intestine of adult humans is abnormal and requires immediate medical attention

3. Chylomicrons are transported directly to the liver via the hepatic portal vein

4. "Blood sugar" refers to the amount of glucose in the blood

5. The tissues that use or store the greatest amount of nutrients in the body are the liver, muscle, adipose, and brain

Multiple Choice

6. The primary site of water absorption is the
   a. Stomach
   b. Small intestine
   c. Large intestine
   d. Rectum

7. The enzymes maltase, sucrase, and lactase are produced by the
   a. Salivary glands
   b. Liver
   c. Pancreas
   d. Small intestine

8. Heartburn is caused by
   a. Release of stomach acid into the small intestine
   b. Failure of the gastroesophageal sphincter to close properly
   c. Consuming an excess of milk and dairy products
   d. Bacterial growth in the stomach

9. Once the body's requirement for amino acids is met, what happens to excess dietary amino acids?
   a. They are excreted in the urine
   b. They are converted to vitamins
   c. They are stored in the liver
   d. They are used for energy in the liver

10. Chyme is a mixture of
   a. Food, hydrochloric acid, and pepsin
   b. Food, hydrochloric acid, and pancreatic enzymes
   c. Food, bicarbonate, and bile
   d. Food, bicarbonate, and pancreatic enzymes

Short Answer

11. Explain why the outside coverings of corn kernels pass through the GI tract undigested

12. Glucose and galactose are absorbed by active transport, whereas fructose is absorbed by facilitated diffusion. Explain why dietary fructose is never completely absorbed

13. Why is it impossible for chewing gum to accumulate in the stomach?

14. A diseased gallbladder can interfere with lipid digestion. Even though the gallbladder's function is to store bile, surgical removal of a diseased gallbladder can restore normal lipid digestion. How is this possible?

Essay

15. You have just eaten an oatmeal chocolate chip cookie. Describe what happens to the cookie as it passes through the gastrointestinal tract. Keep in mind that the cookie contains nutrients from all six nutrient categories

Further Reading

Gibson, G.R. & Roberfroid, M.B. (1995) Dietary modulation of the human colonic microbiota: introducing the concept of prebiotics. *Journal of Nutrition*, **125**, 1401–12.

Guyton, A.C. & Hall, J.E. (1996) *Textbook of Medical Physiology*, 9th ed. W.B. Saunders, Philadelphia.

Jackson, K.A. & Savaiano, D.A. (2001) Lactose maldigestion, calcium intake and osteoporosis in African-, Asian-, and Hispanic-Americans. *Journal of the American College of Nutrition*, **20**(Suppl. 2), 198S–207S.

Kalloo, A.N. & Kantsevoy, S.V. (2001) Gallstones and biliary disease. *Primary Care*, **28**, 591–606.

Klein, S., Cohn, S.M. & Alpers, D.H. (1998) The alimentary tract in nutrition. In: *Nutrition in Health and Disease*, 9th ed. (M.E. Shils, J.A. Olson, M. Shike & A.C. Ross, eds), pp. 605–29. Williams & Wilkins, Baltimore.

Orlando, R.C. (2001) Overview of the mechanisms of gastroesophageal reflux. *American Journal of Medicine*, **111**(Suppl. 8A), 174S–7S.

Rusynyk, R.A. & Still, C.D. (2001) Lactose intolerance. *Journal of the American Osteopathic Association*, **101**(Suppl. 4 Part 1), S10–12.

Schuster, M.M. (2001) Defining and diagnosing irritable bowel syndrome. *American Journal of Managed Care*, **7**(Suppl. 8), S246–51.

Turnbull, G.K. (2000) Lactose intolerance and irritable bowel syndrome. *Nutrition*, **16**, 665–6.

Chapter 6

The Absorptive State

The metabolic events that occur 1–4 hours after eating a meal represent the **absorptive state**, also known as the postprandial state. (The word "prandial" is derived from the Latin word *prandium*, meaning "early dinner.") These events are characterized by the uptake, utilization, and storage of nutrients within cells. Also important during the absorptive state is the release of insulin from the pancreas into the blood as nutrients are being absorbed. Insulin is an essential hormone that promotes the uptake and storage of nutrients in cells by regulating critical chemical reactions. The following section will focus on the energy-containing nutrients—carbohydrate, protein, and fat—and how cells process them in the absorptive state. While all cells have the ability to take up nutrients, the liver, muscle, adipose, and brain capture the majority of nutrients for storage or immediate use. Each tissue performs a specific function during the absorptive period and this will be discussed individually.

Essential Background

❖ Basic human anatomy
❖ Energy-containing nutrients (Chapter 2)
❖ Absorbable products of nutrient digestion (Chapter 5)
❖ Tissue sites of nutrient uptake (Chapter 5)

Topic 6.1

Liver

Key Points

What makes the liver unique with regard to nutrient absorption?
In what form are nutrients absorbed and stored in the liver?
How does insulin regulate nutrient uptake and storage in the liver?

The liver is often considered a **nutrient distribution center** because of its unique position in the body. Water-soluble nutrients entering the blood from the small intestine flow directly to the liver where most are taken up for processing and storage (figure 6.1). When needed, the liver slowly dispenses nutrients such as glucose and fatty acids into the general circulation for distribution to other tissues. In this way, the liver helps to ensure that all tissues receive a constant supply of nutrients between meals.

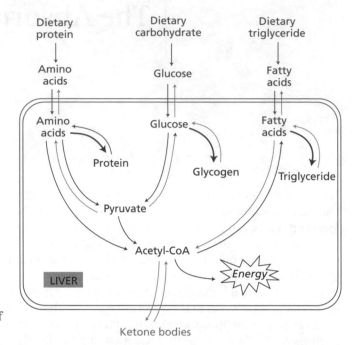

Figure 6.1 Liver metabolism in the absorptive state. The major pathways (bold arrows) are the conversion of dietary amino acids to protein, glucose to glycogen, and fatty acids to triglyceride. Amino acids and glucose are transported directly to the liver via the hepatic portal vein, whereas fatty acids are delivered as chylomicron remnants. These "building" pathways are stimulated by the presence of insulin.

The most abundant dietary carbohydrate entering the hepatic portal vein is glucose, although some fructose and galactose are also present in food and are transported to the liver. About two-thirds of dietary glucose is taken up by liver cells, and the remaining one-third continues on to other tissues. Once inside the liver cell, glucose has three possible fates: (i) conversion to glycogen; (ii) breakdown to yield energy; or (iii) conversion to fatty acids. **Glycogen** is made of glucose molecules linked together to form long chains. The glycogen structure is identical to amylopectin (starch) found in plants except that glycogen is more highly branched, allowing more glucose molecules to attach. The formation of glycogen represents **glucose storage** because the resulting structure is too large to move across the cell membrane. The adult human liver can store about 100 grams of glycogen. While most glucose is stored as glycogen, some incoming glucose is immediately broken down to meet the constant energy needs of the liver. (It is important to note that all tissues have a constant demand for energy to maintain normal function, regardless of a person's dietary state.) Once glycogen storage has reached maximum capacity, excess glucose may be converted to fatty acids for triglyceride synthesis. The triglyceride is then packaged into very low density lipoproteins (**VLDL**) and released into the blood for transport to other tissues, primarily muscle and adipose. (Similar to chylomicrons, VLDL are lipid–protein complexes that allow lipid to be transported in the aqueous bloodstream. The main difference between VLDL and chylomicrons is that VLDL transport fatty acids from the liver to other tissues, whereas chylomicrons transport fatty acids from the small intestine.)

The liver captures virtually all dietary fructose and galactose that enters the blood after intestinal absorption. Galactose is converted to glucose and thus has the same fate as glucose. Conversely, very little fructose is converted to glucose; fructose is either converted to fatty acids for triglyceride synthesis or broken down and used for energy within the liver. Not surprisingly, diets very high in fructose can cause an increase in blood triglyceride levels due to excess triglyceride produced by the liver and released into the blood.

Most dietary fatty acids—transported mainly as triglycerides in chylomicrons—are delivered to adipose and muscle. Once depleted of triglyceride, the chylomicron "remnants" are removed from the circulation by the liver. These leftover components of chylomicrons can be reassembled into VLDL and later released into the blood. Fatty acids are not used for energy in the liver during the absorptive state because the liver's energy needs are met by dietary glucose and excess amino acids.

Some dietary amino acids are taken up by the liver, while the remainder passes through the liver and are transported in the blood to other tissues (figure 6.1). The primary role of amino acids in the liver is to replenish any proteins that were degraded since the last meal. Most of the proteins normally found in circulating blood are made in the liver and released into the blood when needed. Amino acids cannot be stored in the body in the same way that glucose and fatty acids are stored as glycogen and triglyceride. Therefore, excess amino acids in the absorptive state are broken down for energy or converted to fatty acids for triglyceride synthesis.

Of the dietary amino acids entering the liver, the so-called branched chain amino acids (leucine, isoleucine, and valine) tend to escape metabolism and pass through into the general circulation where they are preferentially taken up by muscle. Exercise physiologists are interested in branched chain amino acids because their level in blood tends to decrease with prolonged exercise, triggering the production of serotonin. Because serotonin depresses the central nervous system, decreased levels of branched chain amino acids are thought to be associated with the onset of fatigue. Some researchers have tested the hypothesis that branched chain amino acid supplements can enhance athletic performance, although most studies have generally not supported the hypothesis. Further research is clearly needed to determine if there is truly a link between levels of branched chain amino acids, serotonin, and muscle fatigue.

Insulin is the primary regulator of cellular events during the absorptive period. In the liver cell, insulin signals an increase in glycogen synthesis, fatty acid and triglyceride synthesis, and protein synthesis. Insulin also promotes the conversion of glucose to pyruvate (glycolysis) and acetyl-CoA production. As mentioned in Chapter 3, acetyl-CoA is either converted to fatty acids or used for energy.

Topic 6.2

Muscle

> **Key Points**
>
> What makes muscle unique with regard to nutrient absorption?
> In what form are nutrients absorbed and stored in muscle?
> How does insulin regulate nutrient uptake and storage in muscle?

Two main events occur in muscle during the absorptive period: **glycogen synthesis** and **protein synthesis** (figure 6.2). Insulin signals the muscle cell to take up blood glucose and convert it to glycogen for storage. Adult humans can store up to 400 grams of glycogen in muscle. It is important to note that muscle takes up glucose from the circulation only in the absorptive state when insulin is present; muscle does not remove glucose from blood in postabsorptive or fasting states when insulin is not present.

To maximize their muscle and liver glycogen stores, some athletes engage in **carbohydrate loading**, where specific exercise routines and high-carbohydrate diets are used several days before an athletic event. The method is thought to provide greater energy reserves for individuals engaged in prolonged periods of physical activity, such as distance running or cross-country skiing. A typical protocol begins several days before the scheduled event and involves first depleting the body

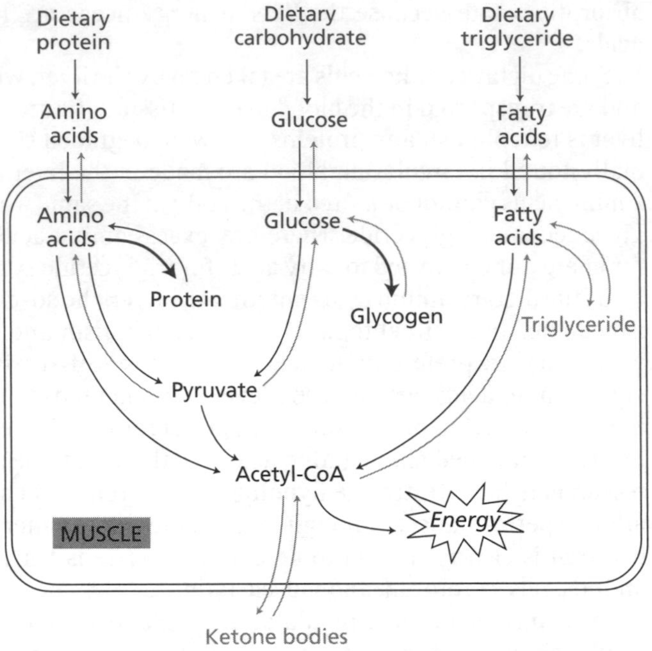

Figure 6.2 Muscle metabolism in the absorptive state. The major pathways (bold arrows) are the conversion of dietary amino acids to protein and the conversion of glucose to glycogen. Muscle also utilizes some fatty acids for energy in the absorptive state, but lacks the ability to convert fatty acids to triglyceride. Insulin stimulates the uptake of amino acids and glucose, and promotes the synthesis of protein and glycogen.

of glycogen stores by exercising. For the next few days, the level of exercise should be tapered while maintaining a moderate carbohydrate diet. Two or three days prior to the event should include low levels of exercise or rest while consuming a high-carbohydrate diet. The amount of dietary carbohydrate should be about 8–10 grams per kilogram of body weight, or about 400–700 grams per day depending on individual size. While this level of carbohydrate is slightly higher than normally recommended for physically active people, drastic changes in dietary habits should be avoided.

Insulin also causes an increase in amino acid uptake and protein synthesis in muscle cells. The primary use of dietary amino acids in muscle in the absorptive state is to **replenish proteins** that were degraded since the last meal. Once the muscle's protein needs are met, excess amino acids may be circulated back to the liver where they are used for energy or converted to fatty acids for triglyceride synthesis. Some of the excess amino acids can be used for energy in the muscle.

Muscle cells can also take up fatty acids from circulating chylomicrons and use them for energy, although dietary glucose is the primary energy source in the absorptive state. Unlike liver and adipose, muscle cells cannot store fatty acids as triglyceride to a great extent.

Topic 6.3

Adipose

Key Points

What makes adipose unique with regard to nutrient absorption?
In what form are nutrients absorbed and stored in adipose?
How does insulin regulate nutrient uptake and storage in adipose?

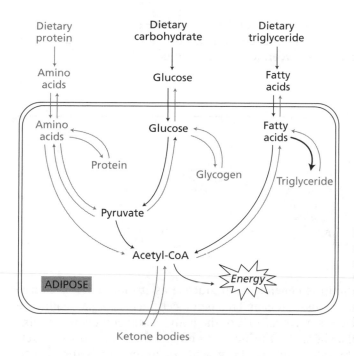

Figure 6.3 Adipose metabolism in the absorptive state. The major pathway (bold arrow) is the conversion of fatty acids to triglyceride for storage. Glucose is also taken up by adipose and provides the energy needed for triglyceride assembly. Fatty acids are delivered to adipose as chylomicrons.

Adipose cells have an almost unlimited ability to synthesize and **store triglyceride**. Consequently, adipose tissue represents the largest energy reserve in the body. In the absorptive state, insulin causes an increase in the uptake of both blood glucose and fatty acids (from chylomicrons). Insulin then promotes the rapid assembly of the fatty acids into triglyceride for storage (figure 6.3). The incoming glucose provides the energy needed for triglyceride assembly, but essentially no dietary glucose is converted to fatty acids in adipose under normal circumstances. Synthesis of fatty acids from glucose in adipose can occur, but only under extreme conditions when a previously starved individual is fed large amounts of carbohydrate.

A common belief among consumers is that carbohydrates will turn into body fat when consumed. In promoting this idea, several diet books such as *Sugar Busters*, *The Atkins Diet*, and *The Zone* have put the blame on carbohydrates for the high incidence of obesity in the United States and urged consumers to reduce their carbohydrate intake. Some books even suggest that certain types of carbohydrate—starch, table sugar, high fructose corn syrup—will effect how much is converted to body fat. The truth is, the ability to make fat from carbohydrate is absent or extremely low in humans under most dietary conditions, even after a large carbohydrate meal. The reason is that carbohydrates are the main energy source for the brain and other tissues that require a constant supply of glucose, so it doesn't make sense that the body would spend energy to chemically convert glucose into fatty acids and then store them as triglycerides in adipose tissue. Furthermore, a fairly large amount of dietary carbohydrate can be stored as carbohydrate (glycogen) in muscle and liver—about 400 and 100 grams, respectively. For example, an adult male who consumes a high-carbohydrate diet (3,000 kcal per day with 60% as carbohydrate) would eat about 450 grams of carbohydrate per day. Notice that the amount of carbohydrate consumed in this generous diet is well within the capacity of muscle and liver to store it as glycogen. So why do people get fat consuming carbohydrates? A body that is in energy balance will burn significant amounts of fat for energy. If there is plenty of carbohydrate around to meet the body's energy needs, then body fat is spared. Consuming a diet that, over the long term, contains more total energy than the body needs means that any incoming dietary fat will go directly to adipose for storage. Excess dietary protein can also be converted to fat and stored in adipose. Therefore, while dietary carbohydrates do not turn into fat, they can contribute to body fat accumulation *when total energy intake exceeds the body's requirements.* Consuming carbohydrates at the recommended amount of 55–60% total kcalories as part of a well-balanced diet does not promote triglyceride storage in adipose tissue.

Topic 6.4

Brain

Key Points

What is the primary energy source used by the brain?
What makes the brain unique with regard to nutrient utilization?

Under normal dietary conditions, the brain is dependent on glucose as its **sole energy source** (figure 6.4). Other tissues of the central nervous system and red blood cells also depend on glucose as their sole energy source. The brain uses as much as 20% of the body's total energy and, unlike muscle, uses energy at a constant rate. Furthermore, the brain has no metabolic means to convert glucose to glycogen for storage. The brain cannot use fatty acids or amino acids for energy. Because of the vital role of the brain in controlling proper body function, a high priority is given to providing the brain with a continual supply of glucose. This is easily achieved in the absorptive state when ample dietary glucose is available. In postabsorptive states, however, glucose must come from other tissues. In starvation or when carbohydrates are lacking in the diet, the brain will adapt to an alternative energy source called ketone bodies (see Chapter 7).

Although the brain uses only glucose for energy under normal circumstances, there is an abundance of so-called health products being sold as "brain fuel" or "brain food." A quick search on the

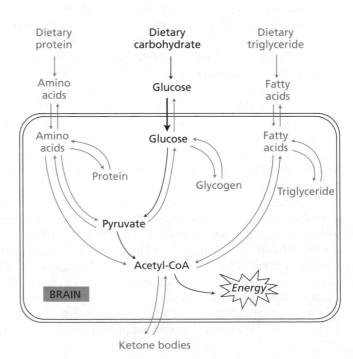

Figure 6.4 Brain metabolism in the absorptive state. The major pathway (bold arrow) is the uptake of blood glucose. The brain lacks the ability to synthesize glycogen and is completely dependent on a constant supply of blood glucose. The brain also lacks the ability to utilize amino acids or fatty acids for energy and depends on glucose as its sole energy source.

internet provides dozens of websites claiming to have products that improve brain power and even reduce the risk of brain disorders such as Alzheimer's disease. Some companies make further claims that scientific studies have proven that their products work. Unfortunately for consumers, most of these products are devoid of carbohydrate and therefore are completely useless with regard to proving energy to the brain. One can also search the scientific literature for studies supporting these claims, but will find that no such studies exist. The notion that you can energize your brain by taking a pill may be a successful advertising ploy, but does nothing for consumers except deplete their wallets. *Caveat emptor . . .* let the buyer beware!

Application

Fructose is found naturally in many fruits and vegetables and in honey, but the major sources of fructose in developed countries are sucrose and high-fructose corn syrups. Fructose currently supplies about 20% of total calories (about 180 grams/day). Clinical disorders related to fructose metabolism can occur if the amount of dietary fructose exceeds the liver's ability to process it. Fructose accumulation causes the liver to make excess uric acid and release it into the blood. Uric acid crystals can form in the fluids surrounding joints, causing inflammation and pain. The clinical terms used to described these conditions are hyperuricemia (elevated uric acid levels) and gout (a type of arthritis). Treatment of gout includes limiting the consumption of fructose-containing foods, although several medications are also available for people in whom dietary therapy is not very effective.

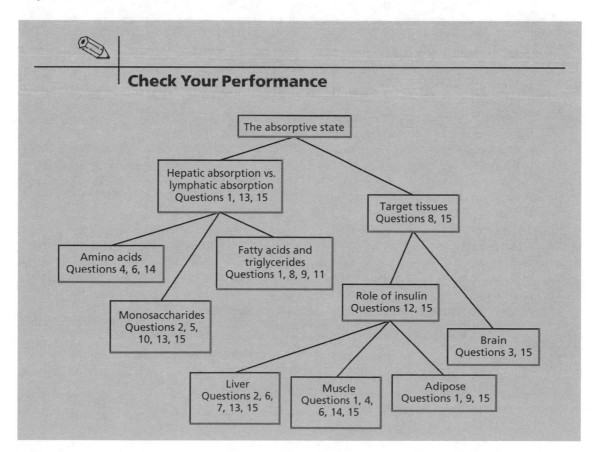

Check Your Performance

Chapter Test

True/False
1. Chylomicrons transport most dietary triglyceride to adipose and muscle
2. Uptake of sucrose by the liver is more efficient than glucose
3. The brain requires significantly less energy during sleep
4. Amino acid accumulation in muscle causes pain and cramping
5. Diets high in fructose can raise blood triglyceride levels

Multiple Choice
6. Excess dietary protein is
   a. Excreted in the feces
   b. Excreted in the urine
   c. Stored in muscle
   d. Used for energy
7. Most of the body's glycogen stores are found in the
   a. Liver
   b. Muscle
   c. Adipose
   d. Brain
8. The primary function of very low density lipoproteins (VLDL) is to
   a. Transport triglyceride from the small intestine to other tissues
   b. Transport triglyceride from the liver to other tissues
   c. Transport triglyceride from adipose to other tissues
   d. Transport triglyceride from muscle to other tissues
9. Excess dietary triglyceride is
   a. Converted to glucose for use by the brain
   b. Stored in the liver
   c. Stored in adipose
   d. Converted to amino acids for use by muscle
10. The common term "blood sugar" refers to
    a. Fructose
    b. Glucose
    c. Sucrose
    d. Amylose

Short Answer
11. Why should you fast overnight before having your blood drawn for triglyceride analysis?
12. What is the main role of insulin in the absorptive state?
13. What happens to dietary galactose after absorption?
14. What is the primary use of amino acids in the absorptive state?

Essay
15. Describe what happens to dietary glucose after it is absorbed into the body. Your discussion should include the major route(s) of glucose in the absorptive state, the sites of tissue uptake, and the fate of glucose once it reaches its destination

Further Reading

Champe, P.C. & Harvey, R.A. (1994) *Lippincott's Illustrated Reviews: Biochemistry*. Lippincott–Raven, Philadelphia.

Felber, J.P. & Golay, A. (1995) Regulation of nutrient metabolism and energy expenditure. *Metabolism*, 44(Suppl. 2), 4–9.

Havel, R.J. (1997) Postprandial lipid metabolism: an overview. *Proceedings of the Nutrition Society*, 56, 659–66.

Shah, M. & Garg, A. (1996) High-fat and high-carbohydrate diets and energy balance. *Diabetes Care*, 19, 1142–52.

Stubbs, R.J., Mazlan, N. & Whybrow, S. (2001) Carbohydrates, appetite and feeding behavior in humans. *Journal of Nutrition*, 131, 2775S–81S.

Watford, M. & Goodridge, A.G. (2000) Regulation of fuel utilization. In: *Biochemical and Physiological Aspects of Human Nutrition* (M.H. Stipanuk, ed.), pp. 384–407. W.B. Saunders, Philadelphia.

Chapter 7

The Fasting State

When no food is consumed, the body must rely on stored nutrients for energy. Which nutrients are used and by what tissues depends largely on how much time has passed since the previous meal. In this sense, the fasting state is not a single state, but rather a continuum of metabolic conditions in which stored nutrients are released into the blood for transport to other tissues for processing or used directly by the tissues in which they are stored. The following discussion will focus on the metabolic events that occur in short-term fasting states (e.g., between meals or sleeping through the night) and long-term fasting states (e.g., starvation or consuming very low calorie diets).

The short-term fasting state—also called the postabsorptive or early fasting state—is the 4–48-hour period following a meal. Consuming another meal will halt the breakdown of stored nutrients, thus ending the short-term fasting state. Consequently, people who consume two or three normal meals as part of their daily routine will cycle between the absorptive and short-term fasting state throughout the day. In addition to stored glucose and fatty acids, the body uses amino acids from muscle protein during the short-term fasting state. The fasting state can become more severe when food is unavailable, when it is voluntarily restricted, or in clinical situations where patients cannot eat. In long-term fasting states greater than 48 hours, the body adapts by reducing its basal metabolic rate and conserving muscle protein. Equally remarkable is the body's ability to produce and use **ketone bodies** as an alternative energy source during long-term fasting states.

Essential Background

❖ The energy-containing nutrients and how they distribute their energy (Chapters 2 and 3)
❖ The role of insulin in nutrient absorption, tissue uptake, and storage (Chapter 6)
❖ Major tissue sites of nutrient storage (Chapters 5 and 6)

Topic 7.1

Liver

Key Points

What are the primary functions of the liver in fasting states?
What major changes occur in short-term versus long-term fasting states?
How does glucagon regulate nutrient breakdown and processing in the liver?

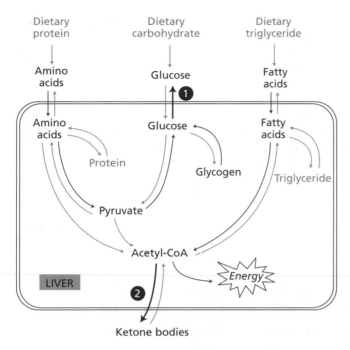

Figure 7.1 Liver metabolism in the fasting states. The major pathway in the short-term fasting state (bold arrow ❶) is the release of glucose into the blood to maintain normal blood glucose concentrations at 70–100 mg/dL. Glucose may come from stored glycogen or by conversion from amino acids via gluconeogenesis. In long-term fasting states, the fatty acid concentration in the blood increases and the liver begins making ketone bodies (bold arrow ❷). By this time, glycogen stores are depleted and gluconeogenesis is shut down to conserve amino acids and body proteins. Fatty acids from adipose provide the main source of energy for the liver in short-term and long-term fasting states.

Short-Term Fasting State

An important goal of the body in short-term fasting states is to maintain **blood glucose** levels at around 70–100 mg/dL so that the brain has a constant and adequate fuel supply. The liver is the primary source of glucose during this time. **Glycogen** stored in the liver is converted back to glucose and released into the blood for transport to the brain and other tissues that rely on glucose as their sole energy source (figure 7.1, ❶). However, liver glycogen stores are limited to about 100 grams and can only replenish blood glucose for a few hours; liver glycogen stores are essentially depleted after an overnight fast. To compensate, the liver can make glucose from amino acids via **gluconeogenesis**. Both gluconeogenesis and conversion of glycogen to glucose are stimulated by the hormone **glucagon**. Muscle protein provides most of the amino acids converted to glucose in the liver. The kidney can also make glucose from amino acids, but the liver accounts for 90% of the glucose made in a short-term fasting state. While it is not desirable to use up muscle protein during long-term fasting situations, short-term use of amino acids for glucose production does not compromise muscle function. Keep in mind that the most important goal is to provide enough glucose for the brain in the absence of dietary carbohydrate. The need to maintain adequate blood glucose levels is so great that the liver does not use glucose for its own energy needs in fasting states; instead, **fatty acids** from adipose are the major source of energy for the liver in short-term (and long-term) fasting states.

Long-Term Fasting State

When food is absent for several days or longer, liver glycogen stores are completely depleted and production of glucose from amino acids is also reduced in an effort to **spare muscle protein**. The overall result is a gradual decrease in blood glucose and decreased glucose availability for energy. The deficiency in glucose causes the body to rely more heavily on fatty acids and their breakdown products—**ketone bodies**—as an energy source. Release of fatty acids from adipose is greatly accelerated in long-term fasting states and fatty acid concentration in the blood is significantly increased. This is fine for tissues that can use fatty acids for energy such as liver and muscle, but the brain cannot use fatty acids. Fortunately, the liver has the ability to convert excess fatty acids to ketone bodies (figure 7.1, ❷). When the concentration of ketone bodies in the blood becomes high enough, the brain and other tissues will start using them for energy. Note that ketone body production and utilization represents a survival mechanism by the body and is not a desirable condition. Increased concentrations of ketone bodies in the blood causes **ketosis** (also called acidosis or ketoacidosis) in which the blood becomes acidic. The effect of prolonged ketosis is depression of the central nervous system, eventually causing coma and death. Individuals who are on starvation diets or who severely restrict their carbohydrate intake (as recommended with many popular "protein" diets) promote ketosis and are at increased risk of developing health problems.

Topic 7.2

Muscle

> ### Key Points
>
> What is the primary role of muscle in fasting states?
> What major changes occur in short-term versus long-term fasting states?
> How does glucagon regulate nutrient breakdown and processing in muscle?

Short-Term Fasting State

Muscle activity accounts for as much as one-third of the total energy used by the body, so a continual supply of energy is needed even between meals. The primary source of energy in the short-term fasting state is **glycogen** stored in muscle (figure 7.2, ❶). The conversion of glycogen back to glucose is stimulated by the hormone **glucagon**. The lack of insulin also prevents the uptake of glucose from the blood, thus conserving blood glucose for use by the brain and other critical tissues that depend on blood glucose. Moreover, muscle glycogen is used only in muscle for energy and is not a source of glucose for the blood. It is important to note that while both muscle and liver store energy as glycogen, the role glycogen plays in these two tissues is quite different. Because muscle glycogen stores are limited and may be depleted within a few hours, a secondary energy source during the short-term fasting state is **fatty acids** from adipose. Fatty acid breakdown in muscle is controlled by **glucagon**. Actually, fatty acids are a steady supply of energy for muscle regardless of whether a person is eating. The relative proportion of energy derived from glycogen versus fatty acids is variable and depends on the intensity and duration of physical activity (see Chapter 14). In addition, some muscle protein is sacrificed during the short-term fasting state to provide amino acids for **gluconeogenesis** in the liver (figure 7.2, ❶).

Long-Term Fasting State

After several days without food, amino acid release into the blood decreases in an effort to conserve muscle mass. This causes the liver to shut down gluconeogenesis and begin making

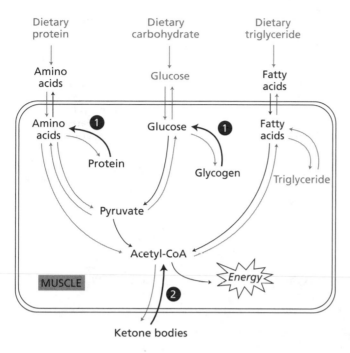

Figure 7.2 Muscle metabolism in the fasting states. The major pathways in the short-term fasting state (bold arrow ❶) are the use of stored glycogen for energy and the release of amino acids into the blood for gluconeogenesis in the liver. In long-term fasting states, muscle adapts to using ketone bodies for energy (bold arrow ❷) when their concentration in blood becomes sufficiently high. Fatty acids from adipose also provide energy for muscle in both short-term and long-term fasting states.

ketone bodies from fatty acids. Consequently, muscle adapts to using ketone bodies for energy when the ketone body concentration in blood becomes sufficiently high (figure 7.2, ❷). Also, muscle continues to use **fatty acids** directly from adipose in long-term fasting states.

Topic 7.3

Adipose

Key Points

What is the primary role of adipose in fasting states?
What major changes occur in short-term versus long-term fasting states?
How is fatty acid release from adipose regulated?

Short-Term Fasting State

The major function of adipose is to provide **fatty acids** for energy when dietary nutrients are absent. (Body fat can also serve as an insulator and as a cushion for internal organs, although these roles are secondary to its role as a critical energy reserve.) Although a small amount of fatty acids are used to meet the energy needs of adipose cells, the majority are released into the blood for transport to other tissues, primarily liver and muscle (figure 7.3). Fatty acids do not easily dissolve in the blood when released from adipose; therefore, they quickly attach to the

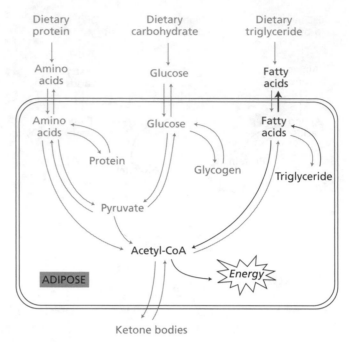

Figure 7.3 Adipose metabolism in the fasting states. The sole purpose of adipose is to provide fatty acids to other tissues for energy (bold arrow). Stored triglycerides are broken down to fatty acids and released into the blood where they bind to the protein albumin for transport to other tissues. A small proportion of fatty acids are used for energy within adipose cells.

protein **albumin** for transport. One albumin molecule can bind several fatty acid molecules for delivery to other tissues. Unlike liver and muscle, adipose is relatively insensitive to the action of glucagon. Two other hormones—**epinephrine** and **norepinephrine**—control the release of fatty acids from adipose.

Long-Term Fasting State

The body becomes increasingly dependent on fatty acids from adipose as an important energy source in long-term fasting states. When the liver decreases the synthesis of glucose from amino acids, release of fatty acids into blood is accelerated, thus increasing the level of circulating fatty acids. The supply of fatty acids exceeds demand in long-term fasting states, causing the liver to convert excess fatty acids into ketone bodies.

In starvation, survival time depends on how much **body fat** a person has prior to fasting. It may be possible for an obese individual to survive several weeks without food, although the ensuing ketosis could be more life threatening than the lack of dietary nutrients. Assuming that ketosis is not too severe, survival time can be estimated.

We know that 1 g of fat provides 9 kcal (kilocalories) of energy; therefore, 1 kg of body fat (2.2 pounds) should theoretically contain 9,000 kcal. In reality, 1 kg of body fat contains only 7,700 kcal because adipose tissue also contains some protein, water, and other metabolic components. Let's assume, then, that a 60-kg (132-pound) person begins a starvation diet with 20% body fat. That means this person has 12-kg of body fat containing 92,400 kcal (12 kg × 7,700 kcal/kg = 92,400 kcal). To maintain basic metabolic functions, the body will require about 1,400 kcal per day—and that does not include any physical activity! Therefore, this person could theoretically live 66 days (less time if the person is physically active) using just body fat stores for energy. It's interesting to note, although somewhat tragic, that several years ago many Irish prisoners starved themselves to death. The average length of survival during starvation was 60 days.

Topic 7.4

Brain

> ## Key Points
>
> What are the primary energy sources for the brain in fasting states?
> What major changes occur in short-term versus long-term fasting states?

Short-Term Fasting State

The brain requires a constant supply of energy to control all of the body's functions. Because the brain cannot store energy as glycogen or triglyceride, it relies on circulating **blood glucose** as its sole source of energy in the short-term fasting state (figure 7.4, ❶). Moreover, the brain cannot use fatty acids or amino acids directly for energy. Through gluconeogenesis, the liver converts amino acids into blood glucose. Most of the glucose produced by the liver during the short-term fasting state is used by the brain, while the rest is used by other tissues that rely on blood glucose as their sole energy source (i.e., red blood cells, retina, and other nervous tissue). Although the hormones insulin and glucagon are not directly involved in brain metabolism, it is still important that insulin is not produced by the pancreas during fasting states. Recall that the presence of insulin promotes the rapid uptake of blood glucose by muscle and adipose, which would leave the brain without its primary energy source.

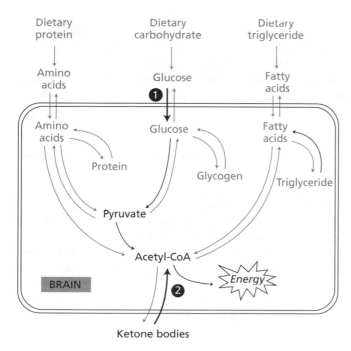

Figure 7.4 Brain metabolism in the fasting states. The brain must receive a constant and steady supply of energy to maintain normal body function. In the short-term fasting state, the brain uses blood glucose as its sole energy source (bold arrow ❶). Blood glucose is replenished in the short-term fasting state by the liver. When blood glucose levels decrease and blood ketone body levels increase, the brain adapts to using ketone bodies for energy (bold arrow ❷).

Table 7.1 Summary of metabolism of insulin and glucagon

Insulin	Glucagon
• Made in β cells of pancreas	• Made in α-cells of pancreas
• Production stimulated by rising blood glucose and amino acids from diet	• Production stimulated by low blood glucose
• Binds to receptors on cell surface of most tissues, but mainly liver, muscle and adipose	• Binds to receptors on cell surface of liver
• ↑ glucose uptake in muscle and adipose	• ↑ glycogen breakdown in liver
• ↑ glycogen synthesis in liver and muscle	• ↓ glycogen synthesis in liver
• ↓ glycogen breakdown in liver	• ↑ gluconeogenesis in liver
• ↓ gluconeogenesis in liver	• ↑ fatty acid breakdown and ketone body synthesis in liver
• ↑ triglyceride synthesis in adipose	• ↑ amino acid uptake in liver for gluconeogenesis
• ↑ amino acid uptake in muscle and most other tissues	
• ↑ protein synthesis in muscle and most other tissues	

Long-Term Fasting State

The brain adapts to using **ketone bodies** for energy when their concentration in the blood becomes markedly elevated (figure 7.4, ❶). While the brain continues to use whatever blood glucose is available in long-term fasting states, the supplemental energy provided by ketone bodies reduces the need for the liver to make glucose at the sacrifice of body protein. In this way, ketone body use by the brain helps to conserve body proteins for other critical functions such as the production of antibodies and enzymes. While the most obvious long-term fasting state is starvation, very low calorie diets that do not meet the body's energy needs can create similar metabolic conditions.

As we have seen, most of the metabolic events that occur in the fasting state are controlled by the hormone **glucagon**. Whereas **insulin** promoted the uptake and storage of nutrients, glucagon has the opposite effect of promoting the breakdown of nutrients for energy and the release of nutrients into the blood for transport to other tissues. Table 7.1 summarizes the metabolic events regulated by insulin and glucagon during the transport, storage, and utilization of the "energy" nutrients.

Application

Low-carbohydrate diets are currently being promoted as a way of losing excess body fat and improving health. These diets, such as Sugar Busters and the Atkins Diet, encourage consumers to limit their intake of carbohydrates and to substitute them with high-protein foods. The theory behind these diets is based on the same metabolic changes that occur in long-term fasting states. Recall that an extended absence of dietary carbohydrate (and total energy) causes blood glucose levels to go down, signaling adipose to release fatty acids at an accelerated rate. On the surface, the theory seems quite sound: the faster fatty acids move out of adipose tissue, the faster body fat disappears. Indeed, one can verify the efficacy of these diets by monitoring the increase in blood ketone bodies (the result of fatty acids flooding the liver). Dr. Atkins actually views increased ketone body production a desirable goal under his diet plan. Although the healthfulness of any diet that intentionally raises blood ketone bodies can be debated, the question arises whether the low-carbohydrate diet plans work because of the absence of carbohydrate *per se* or because the diets are simply low in total energy. Clinical studies have shown that lack of interest in the limited food choices for people on low-carbohydrate, high-protein diets results in low total energy intakes that fail to meet the body's daily energy needs. The promoters of low-carbohydrate diets also like to emphasize that high-carbohydrate diets lead to increased insulin production, which in turn promotes the conversion of carbohydrate (glucose) to fatty acids for storage in adipose. Before insulin can be implicated in promoting body fat accumulation, two key issues need to be addressed. First, conversion of glucose to fatty acids occurs to a significant extent only in the liver, not adipose. Second, while it is possible for liver fatty acids to be transported to adipose as triglyceride in VLDL, this process occurs only when total dietary energy repeatedly exceeds the body's energy requirement. Therefore, diets high in carbohydrate do not promote body fat accumulation when consumed as part of an overall diet that adequately meets energy needs.

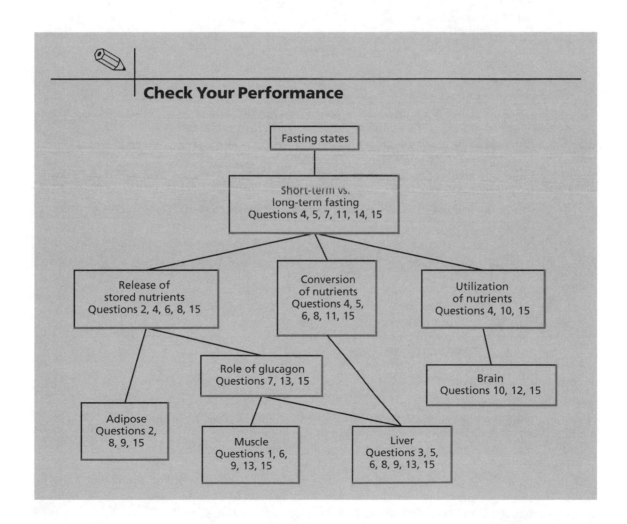

Check Your Performance

Fasting states

Short-term vs.
long-term fasting
Questions 4, 5, 7, 11, 14, 15

Release of
stored nutrients
Questions 2, 4, 6, 8, 15

Conversion
of nutrients
Questions 4, 5,
6, 8, 11, 15

Utilization
of nutrients
Questions 4, 10, 15

Role of glucagon
Questions 7, 13, 15

Brain
Questions 10, 12, 15

Adipose
Questions 2,
8, 9, 15

Muscle
Questions 1, 6,
9, 13, 15

Liver
Questions 3, 5,
6, 8, 9, 13, 15

Chapter Test

True/False
1. Using muscle protein as a source of amino acids for energy is a rare event in humans and only occurs during starvation
2. Fatty acids released from adipose must bind to the protein albumin for transport in the blood
3. Liver glycogen stores are usually depleted by morning after an overnight fast
4. Consumption of very low calorie diets that consistently fail to meet the body's energy needs will produce the same metabolic response as starvation
5. Ketone body production occurs only in the complete absence of food

Multiple Choice
6. After sleeping through the night, what is the most likely source of blood glucose between the time you wake up and before eating breakfast?
    a. Liver glycogen
    b. Muscle glycogen
    c. Amino acids from muscle
    d. Ketone bodies
7. Which of the following hormones is normally absent during fasting states?
    a. Epinephrine
    b. Glucagon
    c. Norepinephrine
    d. Insulin
8. The production of ketone bodies during long-term fasts is due to
    a. Decreased release of glucagon by the pancreas
    b. Increased release of insulin by the pancreas
    c. Increased levels of fatty acids in the blood
    d. Increased levels of amino acids in the blood
9. Which of the following tissues is able to store "energy" for use during fasting states?
    a. Adipose
    b. Muscle
    c. Liver
    d. All of the above
10. The primary goal of the body during fasting states is to
    a. Replenish the glycogen stores in liver and muscle
    b. Provide the brain with a continuous supply of energy
    c. Provide muscle with glucose
    d. Utilize muscle protein as an energy source

Short Answer
11. What causes ketosis?
12. Explain why the presence of insulin would be detrimental to the brain in fasting states
13. What is the difference between glucagon and glycogen?
14. Define "short-term" and "long-term" fasting states

Essay
15. Describe the major metabolic events that occur as an individual goes from the absorptive state to the short-term fasting state to the long-term fasting state

Further Reading

Champe, P.C. & Harvey, R.A. (1994) *Lippincott's Illustrated Reviews: Biochemistry.* Lippincott–Raven, Philadelphia.

Ferraris, R.P. & Carey, H.V. (2000) Intestinal transport during fasting and malnutrition. *Annual Review of Nutrition*, **20**, 195–219.

Ganong, W.F. (2001) *Review of Medical Physiology*, 20th ed. McGraw-Hill/Appleton & Lange, Boston.

Kennedy, E.T., Bowman, S.A., Spence, J.T., Freedman, M. & King, J. (2001) Popular diets: correlation to health, nutrition, and obesity. *Journal of the American Dietetic Association*, **101**, 411–20.

Watford, M. & Goodridge, A.G. (2000) Regulation of fuel utilization. In: *Biochemical and Physiological Aspects of Human Nutrition* (M.H. Stipanuk ed.), pp. 384–407. W. B. Saunders, Philadelphia.

Further reading

Part III

Physiologic Aspects of Nutrition

Chapter 8

Body Composition

The human body is composed of many different types of tissues, each requiring a constant supply of essential nutrients for normal growth and maintenance. Many people in the world struggle to find enough nutrients to meet the body's basic needs, while others enjoy an abundant and diverse food supply. When macronutrients are consumed in excess of the body's need, the excess energy is stored as triglyceride in adipose cells. This process is very efficient and humans have a high capacity to store excess dietary energy as body fat. In nutrition, **body composition** refers to the proportion of fat versus lean with respect to an individual's total body weight. This chapter will address the concept of energy balance and how it is related to body composition. Also presented are strategies that can help maintain a healthy body weight.

Essential Background

❖ Energy capture from the food supply (Chapters 3 and 5)
❖ Storage and use of body fat (Chapters 6 and 7)

Topic 8.1

Energy Balance

> **Key Points**
>
> What is energy balance?
> How is the amount of dietary energy intake determined?
> In what ways does the body expend energy?

If an individual repeatedly consumes more energy than the body needs for growth and normal maintenance, body fat will accumulate. Conversely, consumption of a diet consistently deficient in total energy will result in the loss of body fat as well as lean body mass. **Energy balance** refers to the state in which body weight remains stable because the amount of energy consumed matches the amount used or expended by the body. In other words, **energy in** must equal **energy out** for body weight to remain stable.

Measuring how much energy a person consumes can be easily accomplished with the help of food composition tables and databases. The tables and databases have been developed over a long period of time and are continually being modified as new information is generated regarding the nutrient and energy content of foods. The single most important food composition database is maintained by the US Department of Agriculture. The USDA began publishing the nutrient and energy content of foods in 1896, and now coordinates the most comprehensive system in the world for collecting food composition data. In 1950, the USDA published its famous Handbook No. 8, "Composition of Foods, Raw, Processed, Prepared," that contained at that time information on 15 different nutrients for 751 foods. Handbook No. 8 was expanded many times over the years and was finally computerized in 1991 and released under the new name, "Nutrient Database for Standard Reference." The USDA database has been used by other countries for developing their own nutrient databases, and it serves as the primary starting point for most commercial databases developed by software vendors. Nutrient Database for Standard Reference is also available to consumers via the USDA website (http://www.nal.usda.gov/fnic/foodcomp/).

Commercially available nutrient analysis software is designed to provide the detailed nutrient content of foods. By entering the type and amount of food into the computer, the user can determine, for example, how much vitamin C is in one cup of strawberries. Analysis can be accomplished for single food items or combinations of foods representing several days of consumption. Nutrient analysis software is used most often to estimate an individual's overall dietary pattern for nutrition counseling or medical purposes. Many software companies have developed food analysis systems that are available for consumer and professional use. While most of these software programs start with and build on the USDA nutrient database, significant variation among the programs can exist for several reasons. First, the USDA nutrient database is by no means a complete database, and most nutrient analysis software contains information on hundreds of additional foods for which the vendor must find the nutrient information. The USDA has historically avoided including brandname foods, so most software developers have augmented their databases with brandname foods as well as multiple variations of a single type of food (e.g., "tuna, light, canned in oil" or "tuna, light, canned in water" or "tuna, light, canned in oil, no salt" or "tuna, white, canned in water," etc.). Second, the extent to which the software programs have missing values varies considerably, particularly for foods that are added by the vendors. Third, some software vendors update their databases more frequently than others. Sometimes only a partial list of nutrients is available for a food, so updating often can help fill in missing values as the data become available. Finally, some programs allow the user to adjust the amount of food consumed (portion size), while other programs provide pre-defined portion sizes that may not match the actual amount consumed. When choosing a software program, the main concerns are whether the database contains all of the foods of interest, and whether the database is complete for the nutrients of interest. Also keep in mind that some software programs may be better suited than others for analyzing the diets of certain populations or ethnic groups that consume foods considered unique to that group.

On the other side of the energy balance equation is **energy expenditure**. Humans need energy for three major bodily functions: basal metabolism, physical activity, and the digestion of food. **Basal metabolism** refers to all of the involuntary activities that support life, such as breathing, maintaining body temperature, and pumping of the heart. Basal metabolism accounts for 60–70% of total energy expenditure in most people and can be estimated as 1 kcal/kg of body weight per hour. For an adult female who weighs 58 kg (128 pounds), the **basal metabolic rate** (or **BMR**) needed to support her body's basic functions is estimated to be 1392 kilocalories per day (58 kg × 1 kcal/kg × 24 hours). **Physical activity** accounts for 20–30% of total energy expenditure, although the percentage can be higher depending on the extent of activity. This category includes any muscle movement required for daily life, such as walking, sitting, blinking, or holding a telephone. Energy is also needed for the mechanical and chemical digestion of food. Energy used for this purpose accounts for 5–10% of total energy expenditure and is called the **thermic effect of food**.

Topic 8.2

Body Fat–Too Much, Too Little

> **Key Points**
>
> What problems are associated with too much or too little body fat?
> How is the amount of body fat measured?
> How is the amount of body fat metabolically regulated?

Too much or too little body fat is associated with increased health risks. Problems related to excessive body fat are more common in affluent societies, while too little body fat is more common in underdeveloped countries. But even in economically developed countries, insufficient body fat is often observed in the elderly, people with eating disorders, and people suffering from chronic diseases that inhibit appetite or interfere with eating. In addition to serving as an energy reserve, body fat acts as an insulator in maintaining constant body temperature and helps to cushion internal organs. Insufficient body fat leads to muscle "wasting" because the body must rely on amino acids from muscle protein as a source of energy (see Chapter 7). Too little body fat is also associated with amenorrhea (absence of menstrual cycle), inability to sustain pregnancy, and a decreased ability of the immune system to ward off infection.

Excessive body fat, on the other hand, increases the risk of heart disease, high blood pressure, diabetes, gallbladder disease, stroke, respiratory problems, and certain types of cancer. Because all of these conditions can be life threatening, it is important to health care professionals to define "too much body fat" in clinical terms. **Obesity** is the term used to describe abnormally high amounts of body fat, irrespective of where the excess fat is located in the body. The term **overweight** is also used clinically, but it does not mean the same thing as obesity. Overweight is an increase of body weight relative to a previously defined "desirable" standard. Body weight standards are somewhat arbitrary, but are generally based on the body weight (relative to height) that is associated with lowest mortality (see below). It is possible in some cases—such as body builders—that increased body weight is due to increased amounts of lean muscle mass. However, in the vast majority of people who are overweight, the excess weight is due to increased amounts of body fat and not muscle mass. Despite this potential shortcoming in terminology, "overweight" is used clinically to describe an individual with a body weight of 10–19% above the desirable body weight standard. When body weight is 20% or more above the standard, the individual is classified as "obese."

The concept of a **desirable body weight** was first developed by the life insurance industry more than 100 years ago. In their attempt to find the "most healthy" body weight, insurance companies began compiling data from their policy holders on which body weight categories (relative to height) were associated with the lowest mortality. Eventually weight–height tables were developed that showed the most "ideal" or "desirable" weight. The health care industry later adopted a similar strategy—based on the life insurance weight–height tables—by establishing desirable body weight standards for the general public based on height (table 8.1).

Several methods of assessing body fat are available. The most widely used methods are based on simple body measurements that can be made easily and comfortably. **Body mass index (BMI)** is perhaps the most useful way of comparing weight to height, and is calculated as kilograms/meter^2 (or pounds/inches$^2 \times 704.5$). For example, someone who weighs 59 kilograms (130 pounds) and is

Table 8.1 Body weight ranges corresponding to clinical definitions of desirable weight, overweight, and obese[a]

Height	Desirable weight	Overweight	Obese
4'10"	88–119	120–143	144 and higher
4'11"	91–123	124–148	149 and higher
5'0"	95–127	128–153	154 and higher
5'1"	98–132	133–158	159 and higher
5'2"	101–136	137–163	164 and higher
5'3"	104–140	141–168	169 and higher
5'4"	108–145	146–174	175 and higher
5'5"	111–149	150–179	180 and higher
5'6"	114–154	155–185	186 and higher
5'7"	118–159	160–191	192 and higher
5'8"	121–163	164–196	197 and higher
5'9"	125–168	169–202	203 and higher
5'10"	129–173	174–208	209 and higher
5'11"	132–178	179–214	215 and higher
6'0"	136–183	184–220	221 and higher
6'1"	140–188	189–226	227 and higher
6'2"	144–194	195–232	233 and higher
6'3"	148–199	200–239	240 and higher
6'4"	152–204	205–245	246 and higher
6'5"	156–210	211–252	253 and higher
6'6"	160–215	216–258	259 and higher

[a] Height is measured without shoes, and weight (in pounds) is measured without clothes.
Source: *Dietary Guidelines for Americans* (2000) US Departments of Agriculture and Health and Human Services.

1.7 meters (67 inches) tall has a BMI of 20.4. Although the amount of body fat is not directly assessed using BMI, there is a high correlation between BMI and other methods that measure body fatness. Using this method, normal or desirable weight is usually defined as a BMI of 18.5–24.9; overweight is 25.0–29.9; and obese is 30.0 or greater. Note that these definitions, as used in the Dietary Guidelines for Americans, are designed for educational purposes and a certain amount of judgment needs to be used when assessing a person's health. The biggest limitation of BMI is its inability to directly determine body fat or body fat distribution. **Skinfold thickness** is a method that estimates the amount of fat that lies underneath the skin. Measurements are taken at various locations on the body such as the upper arm, shoulder blade, and waist. Mathematical equations are then used to calculate total body fat. The method is not very accurate and depends on the skill of the technician taking the measurements. Another simple method of estimating body fat is the **waist-to-hip ratio** based on circumference measurements. This method is limited to the body fat around the waist and hip areas, but it is helpful in defining fat distribution. This is important because body fat that is distributed around the waist—but not the hips—is associated with increased risk of heart disease and diabetes. Another method that is sometimes used is **underwater weighing**, in which an individual is weighed both on land and under water. The method is based on the fact that fat is less dense than water, whereas lean body mass is more dense than water. The percentage of body fat can be calculated using mathematical equations that compare both body weights. Underwater weighing is more troublesome and requires specialized equipment. Body composition can also be determined using magnetic resonance imaging (MRI) and computed tomography (CT), but these methods are very expensive and require highly trained technicians to operate the equipment.

One of the greatest mysteries in the field of nutrition is why some people are prone to accumulate body fat while others are not. Clearly, eating more food energy than the body uses is the cause of obesity, but there are poorly understood genetic factors that regulate both appetite and energy expenditure. A child born to obese parents has a significantly greater chance of becoming obese than a child born to normal weight parents, even if the child is raised by adoptive parents. This well-known observation strongly suggests that genetics play an important role in determining a person's body fatness. Several years ago the **set point theory** was developed to help explain how the body tends to settle on a predetermined amount of body fat. When energy intake or physical activity change, the body's metabolism compensates to prevent significant changes in body fat. This may explain why people who lose weight by "dieting" often regain the lost weight, or why thin people have a difficult time gaining weight. The recent discovery of the hormone **leptin** lends support to the set point theory. Leptin is made by fat cells and released into the bloodstream. Consequently, the amount of leptin in the blood depends on how much body fat is present. Studies in animals have shown that circulating leptin signals the brain to decrease appetite and increase energy expenditure. In this way, increased amounts of leptin due to accumulating body fat should help slow the rate at which fat accumulates. However, the role of leptin in humans appears to be more complicated and further research is needed to better understand the contribution of leptin and other genetic factors in determining body fatness.

Topic 8.3

Dieting vs. Weight Management

Key Points

Why do most "diets" fail?
What are the primary attributes of a weight management program?

The balance between energy intake and energy expenditure determines whether a person will gain, lose, or maintain body fat. The concept of energy balance is fairly simple, yet many people living in societies where the food supply is abundant find it difficult to maintain a desirable body weight and, instead, gain excess body fat. In addition to the health consequences, there is a social stigma associated with excess body fat. Overweight individuals are often shunned and discriminated, or at the very least bombarded with advertising that glorifies a thin body. All of these social pressures have driven most overweight individuals to attempt weight loss, usually by restricting the amount of food and energy consumed. The demand for weight-loss programs, dietary supplements, and self-help "diet" books has created a multi-billion-dollar industry that continues to thrive. The success of the weight-loss industry is largely built on the promise that losing excess body fat can be achieved quickly and easily. However, many obesity experts are now questioning whether energy restriction—or so-called **dieting**—is the best approach in view of the fact that the majority of people who lose weight through energy restriction eventually regain the lost weight. Most experts now agree that obtaining a healthy body weight requires more that just short-term weight loss. It requires individuals to view body weight in the context of their overall lifestyle and their ability to maintain a healthy body weight over their lifetime. We refer to this long-term holistic approach as **weight management** to distinguish it from short-term dieting.

One of the major problems with dieting is that it focuses on only one side of the energy balance equation—energy intake. While it is possible to lose weight by restricting energy intake, what happens after the weight has been lost? Unless some change is made in the eating behaviors that caused the weight gain in the first place, it is very likely that the weight will be regained once the dieting phase is completed. **Dieting is not a long-term solution to maintaining a constant and healthy weight.** Unfortunately, most dieting plans available to consumers focus only on short-term weight loss and not on long-term weight management.

Another major problem with dieting is that short-term weight loss is mainly due to losses of **body water**, not body fat. When dietary energy (particularly carbohydrate) is restricted, the body initially relies on glycogen stores for energy. Glycogen in muscle and liver tends to bind water molecules, so when glycogen stores are depleted, water is lost from cells and excreted from the body. The lack of dietary energy also causes some muscle breakdown in order to provide amino acids for glucose synthesis (see Gluconeogenesis, Topics 7.1 and 7.2). Because muscle is composed mostly of water, muscle loss results in water loss. Moreover, the chemical processing of amino acids requires the input of large amounts of body water, causing cells to lose even more water. It is easy to see why energy-restrictive dieting often results in dehydration.

In contrast to dieting, weight management does not necessarily emphasize weight loss as the primary goal. Preventing weight gain and maintaining a stable weight may be more important to good health than losing weight, particularly if someone is losing weight simply to meet a recommended standard or to achieve an unrealistic body image. The most important aspects of long-term weight management are to (i) **avoid dieting** and establish reasonable eating patterns and (ii) **increase physical activity**.

First of all, know that eating is acceptable, normal human behavior; so establishing reasonable eating patterns will help alleviate anxiety about dieting. But it's not always easy to figure out what foods are best for establishing reasonable eating patterns. Thinking about foods in terms of their nutrient and energy content can help emphasize the fact that all foods can fit into a well-balanced diet. To illustrate that there are no "bad" foods or "good" foods (only bad and good diets), consider the classic American cheeseburger. Most people automatically dismiss the cheeseburger as bad for one's health—too much fat, too much sodium, too many calories. But closer inspection reveals that the cheeseburger contains ingredients from every part of the Food Guide Pyramid (page 43) and is really an excellent source of many essential nutrients (figure 8.1). One medium-sized cheeseburger contains 420 kilocalories, 22 grams of fat, and 960 milligrams of

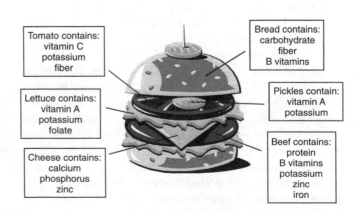

Figure 8.1 Nutrients found in the classic American cheeseburger.

sodium, which is well within recommended daily limit for these nutrients. In fact, even the mayonnaise is an excellent source of vitamin E and essential fatty acids. When viewed from the perspective of nutrient content, it's easier to plan a well-balanced diet that does not necessarily exclude foods we enjoy. Shifting the focus away from the good food/bad food paradigm can help emphasize the more important issues of eating a variety of different foods and limiting portion size. Once again, the Food Guide Pyramid is an excellent resource for thinking in terms of overall diet. It may also be necessary to seek the advice of a registered dietitian in establishing a reasonable eating pattern.

On the other side of the energy balance equation, it helps to find ways of increasing energy expenditure that easily fit into our daily routines. For many people, increasing physical activity could be as simple as taking the stairs instead of the elevator, or parking their car further away from the store's entrance. Any increase in physical activity—however small—will help match energy intake. In this way, long-term weight management over a lifetime of reasonable eating and exercise habits means that some people will experience a reduction in body fat, while others will not. And for many people, this means giving up the fantasy of attaining a super model body that only a fraction of the population will ever achieve. Accepting these realities may not be easy, but the benefits can be long lasting and may help improve one's self-esteem. Also keep in mind that the body weight ranges in Table 8.1 represent average guidelines for the general population and may not be applicable for every individual. Deciding whether to develop a weight management program or to lose weight is a personal decision that should take into account one's current level of body fat, health history, level of fitness, and personal attitude about health and quality of life.

Application

At this very moment, fifty million Americans are dieting despite the overwhelming evidence that diets do not work over the long term. Consumers spend billions of dollars every year on diet books and dieting programs that promise rapid reduction in body fat. Hundreds of diet plans have been published in recent years, including "The Atkins Diet," "The Grapefruit Diet," "The New Pritikin Program," and "The Zone." Virtually all of these diet plans claim that eating certain foods or combination of foods holds the secret to weight loss, or that eliminating certain foods will produce the desired results. The fact that many people are able to lose weight (and sometimes body fat) using these diet plans raises the question of whether specific foods are indeed responsible for promoting weight loss. Close inspection of these diet plans, however, reveals that they all have one thing in common—they are low in total energy. Even The Atkins Diets, which promotes high protein intake, is low in total energy because the lack of food choices and monotony of the diet makes it very difficult to meet the body's daily energy needs. In truth, there are no magical foods that promote fat loss. Diet plans that require consuming special foods or unusual eating times are unlikely to result in spontaneous fat loss from the body. The only way to lose excess body fat is to alter the energy balance equation so that energy expenditure is greater than energy intake.

✎

Check Your Performance

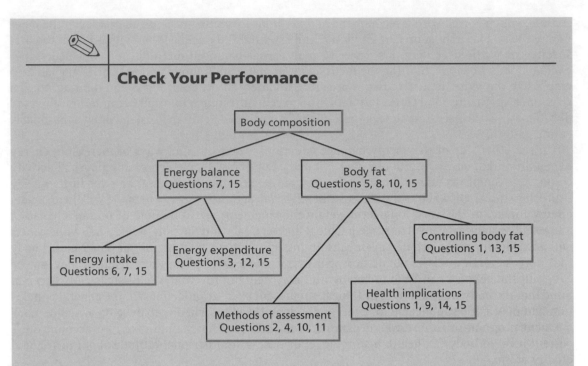

Chapter Test

True/False

1. Weight loss through dieting has long been known to improve health and increase longevity

2. Skinfold thickness measurements are one of the most accurate methods available for determining body fatness

3. "Basal metabolism" refers to all of the involuntary bodily functions that support life, such as breathing and pumping of the heart

4. A person who is 6 feet tall and weighs 170 pounds has a body mass index of 23

5. The belief that every person should achieve a desirable body weight is called the "set point theory"

Multiple Choice

6. The world's most comprehensive system for collecting food composition data is maintained by
   a. The World Health Organization
   b. The Food and Drug Administration
   c. The US Department of Health and Human Services
   d. The US Department of Agriculture
7. Which hormone regulates appetite?
   a. Insulin
   b. Glucagon
   c. Leptin
   d. Growth hormone

8. In nutrition, "body composition" refers to
   a. The proportion of fat versus lean body mass
   b. The percentage of bone mass in the body
   c. The percentage of protein, fat, and minerals in the body
   d. The proportion of body water versus body fat
9. What health problem is not directly associated with excess body fat?
   a. Heart disease
   b. Osteoporosis
   c. High blood pressure
   d. Diabetes
10. Which of the following criteria would classify someone as "obese"?
    a. Body mass index greater than 30
    b. Body weight 10% above the "desirable" weight standard
    c. Waist-to-hip ratio of less than 0.8
    d. All of the above

Short Answer
11. How is underwater weighing able to determine percent body fat?
12. What is the thermic effect of food?
13. What are the major components of a long-term weight management program?
14. Describe the major health problems associated with too little body fat

Essay
15. One of your college friends has a BMI of 28 and has been gradually gaining weight for the past several years. He would like to find a diet plan that will help him lose weight. What would be your advice on how your friend could achieve a more healthy weight?

Further Reading

Astrup, A. (2001) The role of dietary fat in the prevention and treatment of obesity. Efficacy and safety of low-fat diets. *International Journal of Obesity and Related Metabolic Disorders*, 25(Suppl. 1), S46–50.

Blackburn, G.L., Phillips, J.C. & Morreale, S. (2001) Physician's guide to popular low-carbohydrate weight-loss diets. *Cleveland Clinic Journal of Medicine*, 68, 761.

Grundy, S.M. (1999) The optimal ratio of fat-to-carbohydrate in the diet. *Annual Review of Nutrition*, 19, 325–41.

Howarth, N.C., Saltzman, E. & Roberts, S.B. (2001) Dietary fiber and weight regulation. *Nutrition Reviews*, 59, 129–39.

Journal of the American Medical Association (1999) Recent advances in basic obesity research. *JAMA*, 282(16), 1493.

Lee, R.D. & Nieman, D.C. (1996) *Nutritional Assessment*, 2nd ed. Mosby/McGraw-Hill, St Louis.

Lyne, P.A. & Prowse, M.A. (1999) Methodological issues in the development and use of instruments to assess patient nutritional status or the level of risk of nutrition compromise. *Journal of Advanced Nursing*, 30, 835–42.

Lyznicki, J.M., Young, D.C., Riggs, J.A. & Davis, R.M. (2001) Obesity: assessment and management in primary care. *American Family Physician*, **63**, 2185–96.

Rolls, B.J. & Hill, J.O. (1998) *Carbohydrates and Weight Management.* International Life Sciences Institute Press, Washington DC.

Wing, R.R. & Hill, J.O. (2001) Successful weight loss maintenance. *Annual Review of Nutrition*, **21**, 323–41.

Chapter 9

Nutrition-Related Diseases

Diet has long been known to influence chronic diseases, but only in recent years have scientists begun to understand the metabolic basis of disease and the role of specific dietary components. Presented in this chapter is a brief introduction to several major chronic diseases in which diet plays a regulatory role. Coronary heart disease and stroke are discussed together because of their similar metabolic processes and because they appear to be influenced by the same dietary factors. Cancer, hypertension, and diabetes mellitus are also discussed. These five diseases account for more than half of all deaths in the United States and are the primary targets of current dietary recommendations. Osteoporosis, though not always fatal, is the main cause of hip fracture in the elderly and certainly has health implications for much of the elderly population. It is important to recognize that genetic factors and family history are also major determinants of chronic disease, although the role of genetics will not be discussed in this chapter.

Essential Background

❖ Dietary recommendations (Chapter 4)
❖ Normal nutrient metabolism (Chapters 5–7)
❖ Dietary and other lifestyle factors contributing to obesity (Chapter 8)

Topic 9.1

Coronary Heart Disease and Stroke

> **Key Points**
>
> What is coronary heart disease and stroke?
> How is diet related to coronary heart disease and stroke?
> What strategies are thought to reduce the risk of coronary heart disease and stroke?

Cardiovascular disease is a general term that refers to any disease of the heart and circulatory system. Of these, **coronary heart disease** (CHD) and **stroke** account for about 20% and 7% of all deaths in the United States, respectively. Figure 9.1 shows the death rate for CHD and stroke during the last two decades. CHD and stroke are really the same disease, except that they occur in different locations in the body. Both diseases are characterized by the accumulation of fatty material on the inside wall of arteries, which can eventually impede the flow of blood. The process of lipid

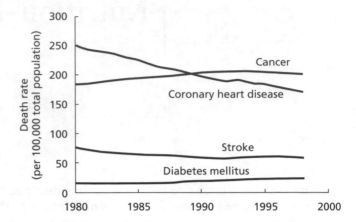

Figure 9.1 Death rate in the United States for cancer, coronary heart disease, stroke, and diabetes mellitus. Source: Centers for Disease Control and Prevention, National Center for Health Statistics.

accumulation is called **atherosclerosis** (or hardening of the arteries), and the lesions that develop are called **plaques**. Atherosclerosis usually begins as a soft "fatty streak" along the inner wall of arteries, especially at branch points. The fatty streaks gradually enlarge and become hardened plaques that damage artery walls, making the walls inelastic and narrowing the passage through them. When a plaque ruptures, the body senses an "injury" and initiates a blood clot to repair the damage. Unfortunately, the blood clot can completely stop the flow of blood in the narrow passageway. When this occurs in an artery that feeds the heart muscle, the abrupt lack of oxygen will cause a heart attack. Blockage in the arteries that lead to the brain will result in a stroke. The severity of a heart attack or stroke depends on the extent of blockage and the amount of tissue that is deprived of oxygen.

Nearly every adult who lives in developed countries has some degree of plaque build up in their arteries. Studies have shown that even teenagers have early signs of atherosclerosis and that most people have well-established plaques by the time they are 30 years old. However, not everyone will suffer the ill effects of a heart attack or stroke. That's because the rate of atherosclerosis and plaque development is different in every person. The question is not whether you have plaque, but rather how far advanced it is and what you can do to slow its progression.

Researchers have identified a number of **risk factors** that are associated with CHD and stroke. Some risk factors such as age and being male are unavoidable, but other risk factors such as smoking, diabetes, lack of exercise, hypertension, elevated serum cholesterol, and obesity can be controlled. Central obesity—body fat accumulation around the abdominal area—is also a risk factor because it can cause diabetes, hypertension, and elevated serum cholesterol levels. Most experts agree that an individual can lower his or her risk for CHD or stroke by changing these risk factors. It's important to recognize that many of these risk factors are directly influenced by an individual's diet.

Hypertension can also be fatal independent of its role in CHD and stroke. Therefore all adults should have their blood pressure checked regularly and strive for a target of less than 140/90 mmHg (systolic/diastolic measurements in millimeters of mercury). Blood pressure readings above these values for either the systolic or diastolic measurement would indicate hypertension. For most people, increased physical activity, weight reduction, restricted alcohol use, and a balanced diet that provides adequate nutrients help to keep blood pressure normal. For some, sodium restriction is also required, although the proportion of adults who are sensitive to dietary sodium is only about 10–15% of the population. A diet low in fat and rich in fruits, vegetables, and whole grains may help to lower blood pressure.

Table 9.1 Dietary recommendations for reducing serum cholesterol concentration

Nutrient	Recommended intake as percent of total calories	
	Step I diet	Step II diet
Total fat	30% or less	30% or less
Saturated	7–10%	Less than 7%
Polyunsaturated	Up to 10%	Up to 10%
Monounsaturated	Up to 15%	Up to 15%
Carbohydrate	55% or more	55% or more
Protein	Approximately 15%	Approximately 15%
Cholesterol	Less than 300 mg per day	Less than 200 mg per day
Total calories	To achieve and maintain desired weight	To achieve and maintain desired weight

Of all the controllable risk factors for CHD and stroke, most attention has focused on serum cholesterol. The goal of many public education programs is to reduce serum cholesterol levels to less than 200 milligrams per deciliter. While several factors control serum cholesterol levels, recommendations generally focus on making dietary changes. In the 1980s, the American Heart Association and the National Cholesterol Education Program (part of the National Institutes of Health) teamed up to develop specific dietary recommendations for individuals with elevated cholesterol levels. The recommendations were established on two levels: the **Step I Diet** is designed to help individuals with moderately elevated cholesterol levels, whereas the **Step II Diet** is more restrictive and is intended to produce greater reductions in blood cholesterol (table 9.1). The main difference between the two diets is the recommended amounts of dietary saturated fat and cholesterol. The use of these diets has been generally successful, although a major limitation is that many consumers don't understand how to calculate how much each nutrient class is contributing to the total energy intake of their diet. In response, the American Heart Association has recently revised the guidelines to put more emphasis on foods and food groups, rather than relying on the percent of food components. The terms "Step I" and "Step II" have also been dropped, but the guidelines still retain the stepwise approach to managing blood cholesterol levels through diet.

The Dietary Guidelines for Americans and Healthy People 2010 (see Topic 4.2) also recommend limiting total fat, saturated fat, and cholesterol intake as a way of reducing serum cholesterol. (It should be noted that the most recent scientific evidence shows that dietary cholesterol has little impact on serum cholesterol levels, although public health officials are reluctant to change this recommendation and it is still included in most public education programs.) Other dietary recommendations include increasing consumption of whole grains, fruits, vegetables, and oily fish rich in omega-3 fatty acids. Regular physical activity and reduction in excess body fat can also lower serum cholesterol. Drug therapy is available for people in whom serum cholesterol levels do not respond to diet or exercise. However, managing serum cholesterol levels through diet and exercise should be the first approach under most circumstances—all drugs have side effects and their use should always be the last resort. While elevated serum cholesterol is an important risk factor for CHD and stroke, other risk factors may be more important in some people. The facts that "normal weight" individuals have heart attacks and that about 40% of deaths from CHD occur in people with serum cholesterol levels below 200 mg/dL suggest that genetics (family history) play an important role.

Topic 9.2

Cancer

> **Key Points**
>
> What is cancer?
> How is diet related to cancer?
> What strategies are thought to reduce the risk of cancer?

One out of every three people in the United States will develop **cancer** in their lifetime. Because the death rate from CHD has been declining in recent years, cancer is now the leading cause of death in the United States, accounting for about 23% of all deaths (figure 9.1). The term "cancer" refers to a group of conditions characterized by the uncontrolled growth of cells arising from almost any tissue of the body. Cancer of the lung, colon and rectum, breast, prostate, and skin occur most frequently. Death due to lung cancer has increased significantly during the past few decades and is now the leading cause of cancer death in both males and females (figure 9.2). Most experts attribute this phenomenon to the high rate of smoking in the United States. By contrast, the death rate

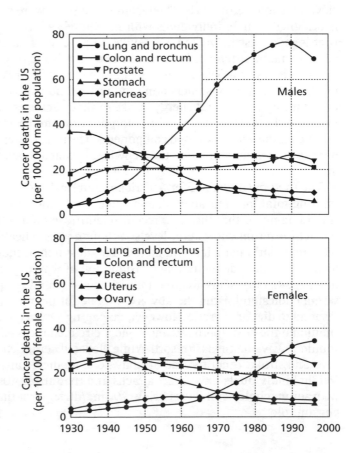

Figure 9.2 Cancer deaths in the United States. Source: Centers for Disease Control and Prevention, National Center for Health Statistics.

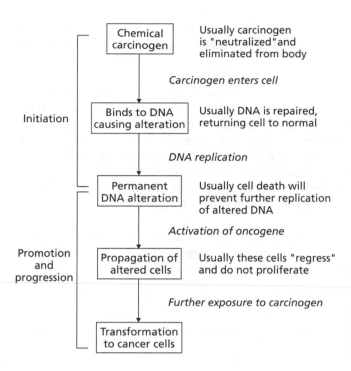

Figure 9.3 Current understanding of chemical carcinogenesis. In addition to chemical induction, oncogenes may be activated by viruses, radiation, hormones, immune conditions, and inherited genetic mutations.

due to stomach cancer in males and uterine cancer in females has declined. Colorectal, prostate, and breast cancer continue to be major causes of cancer death in the United States.

Cancer is caused by both external factors (chemicals, viruses, and radiation) and internal factors (hormones, immune conditions, and inherited genetic mutations). Figure 9.3 illustrates the traditional view of how an external chemical carcinogen causes cancer. First, the chemical carcinogen enters the body through diet, respiration, or absorption through skin and eventually gains entry into a cell. This is the beginning of the **initiation** phase. Most of the time, carcinogens that enter cells are neutralized and excreted from the body, although occasionally a carcinogen will persist and eventually bind to the cell's DNA, altering its genetic structure. At this point the cell can repair the DNA; however, repeated exposure can overwhelm the cell's ability to repair itself and permanent DNA damage can result. But because the altered DNA is not normal, the cell usually dies, thus protecting the body from further abnormalities. If the altered DNA persists long enough, however, a portion of the DNA called an **oncogene** is activated, triggering replication of more altered DNA and increasing the number of abnormal cells. This phase is called **promotion**. Oncogenes are thought to be activated only after several years of repeated exposure to a carcinogen or by the other external or internal factors mentioned above. Finally, the uncontrolled growth of these altered cells results in their transformation to full cancer cells, thus leading to the growth of a new tissue called a **neoplasm** or **tumor**.

Scientists have estimated that about one-third of all human cancer may be caused by carcinogens present in foods we eat. Our bodies are equipped to handle tiny doses of carcinogens that occur naturally in foods. However, repeated exposure at high levels can overwhelm the body's ability to handle the naturally occurring carcinogens. Thus, the best plan for reducing the risk of certain cancers is to minimize exposure to suspected carcinogens and commit to a long-term healthful diet. It is known that foods cooked at high temperature and charcoal broiled foods contain carcinogens called **polycyclic aromatic hydrocarbons** (PAH). Some foods, particularly those preserved with sodium nitrite such as cured meats, contain carcinogens called **nitrosamines**, and many plant foods contain naturally occurring carcinogens. While research has shown that these chemicals—given at high doses—cause cancer in laboratory animals, there is little evidence to indicate that occasional consumption at the relatively low levels found in the food supply will cause human cancer.

Other dietary factors are believed to be **promoters** and **inhibitors** of certain cancers. High-fat diets, particularly those rich in omega-6 fatty acids, are associated with cancer promotion, whereas omega-3 fatty acids appear to have an inhibiting effect. Sucrose consumption promotes cancer, whereas intake of starch and fiber inhibit cancer. Although associations between cancer and dietary fats and carbohydrates have been observed in some studies, the findings are not always consistent. Perhaps the most consistent finding is the inhibitory effect of diets rich in fruits, vegetables, and whole grains. Populations that consume ample amounts of these foods generally have low rates of cancer. Fruits, vegetables, and whole grains are rich sources of fiber, vitamin C, vitamin E, beta-carotene, and many other micronutrients and phytochemicals that appear to offer the best possible protection against cancer promotion.

Although the causes of cancer are not fully understood, scientists are learning more each day. It has been said that cancer, more than any other chronic disease, best illustrates the importance of one of the guiding principles in nutrition: "Balance, variety, and moderation."

Topic 9.3

Diabetes Mellitus

> ### Key Points
>
> What is diabetes mellitus?
> How is diet related to diabetes mellitus?
> What strategies are thought to reduce the risk of diabetes mellitus?

Diabetes mellitus—commonly called "diabetes"—is actually several disorders that are characterized by elevated blood glucose concentration or **hyperglycemia**. Long-term complications associated with hyperglycemia include blindness, kidney failure, nerve degeneration, and circulatory disorders that can lead to amputation of the lower extremities. The main reason why hyperglycemia develops in diabetes is that the glucose in blood is unable to move into cells where it is needed for energy metabolism. This occurs because: (i) the hormone **insulin**, which is required for glucose transport into cells, is not produced by the pancreas or it is produced in insufficient amounts, or (ii) the body's cells have become insensitive to insulin and are therefore unable to accept glucose. Chapters 6 and 7 describe how insulin functions under normal metabolic conditions. In this section, we will discuss two types of diabetes; insulin-dependent and non-insulin-dependent diabetes.

Insulin-dependent diabetes mellitus (IDDM), also called **Type 1** diabetes, accounts for about 10% of all diabetes cases. It was formerly known as **juvenile-onset** diabetes because the majority of patients with IDDM develop the condition in childhood. Initial symptoms of IDDM include increased thirst, increased urination, dehydration, weight loss, blurred vision, and fatigue. In severe cases ketosis may occur (see Chapter 7 for a description of ketosis). IDDM is caused by a deficiency of insulin due to an autoimmune process that destroys the cells in the pancreas that make insulin. People with IDDM are completely dependent on routine insulin injections to prevent hyperglycemia, ketosis, and death. **Non-insulin-dependent diabetes mellitus** (NIDDM), or Type 2 diabetes, accounts for about 90% of all diabetes cases. Previously known as **adult-onset** diabetes (most cases develop after 30 years of age), this term is no longer used because of the increasing incidence of NIDDM in children and young adults. NIDDM is characterized by a combination of insulin resistance and decreased insulin production. Patients with NIDDM are not absolutely dependent on insulin injections and they generally do not develop ketosis. There are several factors related to the onset of NIDDM, but the main factors are obesity, advancing age, and physical inactivity. In fact, about 80% of people with NIDDM are obese.

Diet plays an important role in NIDDM to the extent that reduction in body fat and increased physical activity improves insulin sensitivity and reduces hyperglycemia. Therefore, people with NIDDM should follow the Food Guide Pyramid and dietary guidelines that have been established for the general population, but with special emphasis on total energy balance and weight management. Of course, preventing obesity in the first place with regular exercise and a well-balanced diet is the best strategy for avoiding NIDDM altogether. Nutritional therapies for people with IDDM also focus on well-balanced diets that meet the body's nutrient requirements. However, because people with IDDM must receive insulin injections and monitor their blood glucose very closely, diets that minimize large fluctuations in blood glucose are most useful.

At present there is no single "diabetic diet" that is appropriate for all diabetics, although foods or combinations of foods that have a low **glycemic index** are desirable. Most foods cause blood glucose levels to rise following a meal. Different foods, however, have varying effects on how quickly and by how much blood glucose rises. The glycemic index is a measurement used to describe the effect of specific foods on blood glucose levels. It is a numeric scale that ranks foods in comparison to a reference food. Tables that list the glycemic index of food use either white bread or a glucose solution as the standard, which is arbitrarily set at 100. The glycemic index concept was originally developed to aid health care providers and patients in managing diabetes through dietary means. Foods with a low glycemic index indicate a slower and/or lower rise in blood glucose and would therefore be more desirable (table 9.2). Although generally useful, the glycemic index is limited because it is difficult to predict the blood glucose response when several foods are consumed at the same time as part of a meal. Nevertheless, the increasing number of people—particularly children—with NIDDM has triggered an increased use of glycemic indexes. While tables listing the glycemic index of foods are available to consumers, dietary strategies for the management of diabetes should be developed on an individual basis with the help of qualified health care professionals.

Topic 9.4

Osteoporosis

Key Points

What is osteoporosis?
How is diet related to osteoporosis?
What strategies are thought to reduce the risk of osteoporosis?

Osteoporosis is a degenerative disease characterized by excessive loss of bone minerals, particularly calcium. Osteoporosis is a "silent" disease and usually goes undetected until a bone fracture

Table 9.2 Glycemic index of selected foods

	Glycemic index
Corn flakes	119
Waffles	109
Bagel, white	103
Carrots	101
White bread	**100**
Potatoes	100
Shredded wheat	99
Soft drink	97
Ice cream	87
Blueberry muffin	84
Rice, white long-grain	81
Popcorn	79
Oatmeal	79
Banana	76
Baked beans	69
Orange	62
All-Bran breakfast cereal	60
Spaghetti noodles	59
Apple	52
Yogurt	47
Milk, skim	46
Milk, full-fat	39
Peanuts	21

occurs. It affects about 25 million people in the United States and results in about 1.5 million bone fractures each year. More women are affected by osteoporosis than men, with the highest prevalence occurring after menopause.

To understand the development of osteoporosis, it is helpful to distinguish the differences between **trabecular** and **cortical** bone. Trabecular bone is honeycomb-like bone found in the pelvis, vertebrae, and at the end of long bones. It is metabolically more active than cortical bone and readily gives up calcium to the bloodstream when the blood calcium concentration drops too low. Cortical bone is more dense and does not give up calcium as freely as trabecular bone; consequently, trabecular bone is more easily affected by osteoporosis. The slow loss of calcium over time can also cause the vertebrae to compress into wedge shapes, resulting in curvature of the spine called **kyphosis** or "Dowager's Hump." Compression of the vertebrae can result in the loss of 3–6 inches in height.

Clinical definitions of osteoporosis include two types. **Type I** (or postmenopausal) osteoporosis occurs in women when estrogen levels decline after menopause. Type I osteoporosis occurs mainly in the vertebrae and radius (wrist). With Type I osteoporosis, women lose mostly trabecular bone and fractures become more frequent after age 65. Trabecular bone often becomes so fragile that a woman's body weight can be enough to cause bone fracture of the vertebrae. In **Type II** (or age-related) osteoporosis, demineralization occurs in trabecular and cortical bone, and represents the inevitable loss of bone mass that occurs with age in both men and women. Type II osteoporosis is characterized by demineralization of the vertebrae, hip and pelvis, humerus (upper arm), and tibia (lower leg).

What actually causes osteoporosis is not fully understood, although many factors associated with osteoporosis have been identified. The female hormone **estrogen** promotes bone formation, so the risk of osteoporosis increases dramatically after menopause. **Testosterone** may play a similar role in bone health in men. **Smoking** tends to decrease estrogen levels and therefore contributes to bone loss. **Weight-bearing exercise** has a positive influence on bone mineralization; walking may be better than swimming with regard to bone strength. But perhaps the most important factors contributing to osteoporosis are insufficient amounts of dietary **calcium** and **vitamin D**.

Adequate calcium intake is important throughout life, although it is particularly critical during the growing years when bone density can be optimized. The Dietary Reference Intake for calcium is 1,300 mg per day for both males and females 9–18 years of age. Adequate vitamin D is also critical because it promotes the absorption of dietary calcium from the gastrointestinal tract. Fortifying milk with vitamin D, which is not naturally present in milk, was a logical decision because milk is a natural source of calcium. You should first try to get calcium and vitamin D from food; however, if your food choices do not provide adequate amounts, then calcium and vitamin D supplements may be an appropriate second choice. Calcium supplements are available in three forms: (i) purified calcium compounds such as calcium carbonate, calcium citrate, calcium lactate, calcium malate, calcium phosphate, and calcium gluconate, or compounds of calcium with "amino acids chelates;" (ii) mixtures of calcium with other compounds such as magnesium carbonate, aluminum salts (antacids), or with vitamin D; and (iii) powdered calcium-rich materials such as bone meal, powdered bone, oyster shell, or dolomite (limestone).

Application

The three leading causes of death in the United States—cancer, coronary heart disease, and stroke—are influenced by what we eat. Scientists have even begun to explain the metabolic basis for these and many other chronic diseases. But simply knowing that a relationship exists between diet and disease does not always help people understand their personal risk or chance of developing a disease. Many uncertainties quickly come to mind: How do I know my current diet is unhealthy? What should I change about my diet? And how do I know that changing my diet will be beneficial? These issues are complicated by the fact that genetic factors in some people may be a stronger influence in disease development than diet. As we sort through these issues, it's important to recognize that no one can know with absolute certainty whether they will develop a disease later in life. But by making even small changes in our diet, we just might increase our chances of preventing—or at least delaying—certain chronic diseases. Evidence suggests that dietary and lifestyle changes don't have to be dramatic in order to make a difference in a person's well being. For example, eating smaller portions ("super sizing" is not really necessary) is fairly easy to do and it can help a person stay in energy balance. The fact that 55% of Americans are overweight, and because excess body fat is a risk factor for so many chronic diseases, strongly suggests that controlling total energy intake may be one of the most important dietary changes a person could make. Reducing total fat and saturated fat intake, increasing consumption of high fiber foods, and increasing physical activity may take more planning, but such changes will increase the chance of avoiding chronic disease and may even improve a person's overall health and well being.

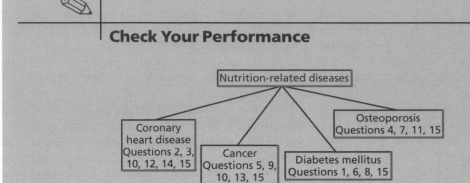

Check Your Performance

Chapter Test

True/False

1. The hallmark of all types of diabetes is severe ketosis
2. Coronary heart disease is the leading cause of death in the United States
3. Most people living in developed countries have some degree of atherosclerotic plaque build up in their arteries
4. Swimming is one of the best types of exercise to increase bone strength
5. It is estimated that about one-third of all human cancer may be caused by carcinogens present in foods we eat

Multiple Choice

6. The most appropriate recommendation for managing non-insulin-dependent diabetes mellitus is to
 a. Reduce excess body fat
 b. Increase physical activity
 c. Follow the Food Guide Pyramid
 d. All of the above
7. The Dietary Reference Intake of calcium for growing children 9–18 years of age is
 a. 300 mg/day
 b. 800 mg/day
 c. 1,000 mg/day
 d. 1,300 mg/day
8. What metabolic condition is common among every type of diabetes?
 a. Elevated blood cholesterol
 b. Elevated blood glucose
 c. Dehydration
 d. Fatigue/muscle weakness
9. Cancer can be caused by each of the following *except*
 a. Radiation
 b. Viruses
 c. Hypertension
 d. Inherited genetic mutations

10. Which of the following is *not* a major cause of death in the United States?
   a. Influenza
   b. Stroke
   c. Cancer
   d. Coronary heart disease

Short Answer
11. Why is trabecular bone more susceptible to osteoporosis than cortical bone?
12. How does obesity increase the risk of coronary heart disease and stroke?
13. Despite routine exposure to chemical carcinogens in our environment, most people never develop cancer. Why?
14. What causes a heart attack?

Essay
15. Discuss in detail how the various risk factors mentioned in this chapter contribute to chronic disease

Further Reading

Aronne, L.J. (2001) Treating obesity: a new target for prevention of coronary heart disease. *Progress in Cardiovascular Nursing*, 16, 98–106, 115.

Atkinson, S.A. & Ward, W.E. (2001) Clinical nutrition: 2. The role of nutrition in the prevention and treatment of adult osteoporosis. *Canadian Medical Association Journal*, 165, 1511–14.

Brown, J., Byers, T., Thompson, K., Eldridge, B., Doyle, C. & Williams, A.M. (2001) Nutrition during and after cancer treatment: a guide for informed choices by cancer survivors. *CA Cancer Journal for Clinicians*, 51, 153–87.

Krauss, R.M., Eckel, R.H., Howard, B., *et al.* (2000) AHA Dietary Guidelines: revision 2000. A statement for healthcare professionals from the Nutrition Committee of the American Heart Association. *Circulation*, 102, 2284–99.

Miller, G.D., Jarvis, J.K. & McBean, L.D. (2001) The importance of meeting calcium needs with foods. *Journal of the American College of Nutrition*, 20(Suppl. 2), 168S–85S.

Morgan, J., Sharma, S., Lukachko, A. & Ross, G. (1999) The breast cancer prevention diet by Dr. Bob Arnot: unscientific and deceptive—a disservice to American women. *Journal of Health Communication*, 4, 235–48.

New, S.A. (2001) Exercise, bone and nutrition. *Proceedings of the Nutrition Society*, 60, 265–74.

Nuttall, F.Q. & Chasuk, R.M. (1998) Nutrition and the management of type 2 diabetes. *Journal of Family Practice*, 47(Suppl. 5), S45–53.

Obarzanek, E., Sacks, F.M., Vollmer, W.M., *et al.* (2001) Effects on blood lipids of a blood pressure-lowering diet: the Dietary Approaches to Stop Hypertension (DASH) Trial. *American Journal of Clinical Nutrition*, 74, 80–9.

Palumbo, P.J. (2001) Glycemic control, mealtime glucose excursions, and diabetic complication in type 2 diabetes mellitus. *Mayo Clinical Proceedings*, 76, 609–18.

Reddy, B.S. (1999) Role of dietary fiber in colon cancer: an overview. *American Journal of Medicine*, 106(1A), 16S–19S.

Robertson, J.I. (2000) The modern treatment of hypertension. *Journal of Human Hypertension*, 14(Suppl. 1), S51–62.

Rose, D.P. (1997) Dietary fat, fatty acids and breast cancer. *Breast Cancer*, 4, 7–16.

Slavin, J.L., Jacobs, D., Marquart, L. & Wiemer, K. (2001) The role of whole grains in disease prevention. *Journal of the American Dietetic Association*, 101, 780–5.

Weisburger, J.H. (2000) Prevention of cancer and other chronic diseases worldwide based on sound mechanisms. *Biofactors*, 12, 73–81.

Young-Hyman, D., Schlundt, D.G., Herman, L., De Luca, F. & Counts, D. (2001) Evaluation of the insulin resistance syndrome in 5- to 10-year-old overweight/obese African-American children. *Diabetes Care*, 24, 1359–64.

Chapter 10

Nutrition Throughout the Life Cycle

All humans require the same nutrients for growth, development, and maintenance of the body's functions. But the amount we need is different for each stage of life. This chapter focuses on the changes that occur in the body during the lifespan and how these changes influence our nutrient and energy requirements. The first section focuses on the special needs of pregnant women and those who choose to breast-feed. Also discussed are the nutritional concerns of growing children and the changes that occur throughout adulthood.

Essential Background

❖ Dietary recommendations at each stage of life (Chapter 4)
❖ Energy balance and weight management (Chapter 8)
❖ Effects of nutrition on disease development (Chapters 4 and 9)

Topic 10.1

Pregnancy and Lactation

> **Key Points**
>
> What physiological changes occur during pregnancy?
> What special dietary concerns are faced by pregnant and lactating women?
> In what ways do infant formula and breast milk differ?

Pregnancy is a time of tremendous change in a woman's body. The nutrient demands of the developing fetus require a mother to make healthful dietary and lifestyle choices that will help ensure a successful pregnancy. An unborn baby is completely dependent on its mother for providing the essential nutrients needed for proper growth and development. Nutrients and oxygen pass from the mother's blood to the baby's in exchange for waste products and carbon dioxide. Although the maternal and fetal blood systems do not actually mix, they are so closely tied that just one bite of spicy food can cause the fetus to kick and move in a most disagreeable manner. More serious concerns, such as nutrient deficiencies or alcohol and drug use, can cause premature births, low birth weights, and birth defects. Following a healthful diet during pregnancy is extremely important, but so is the nutritional health of the mother prior to conception. Fetal development of the brain, arms and legs, eyes, and heart occurs mainly in the first few weeks of life when many women have not

Table 10.1 Guidelines for weight gain during pregnancy

Prepregnancy BMI (kg/m²)	Weight gain (pounds)
Low (<19.8)	28–40
Normal (19.8–26.0)	25–35
High (>26.0–29.0)	15–25
Obese (>29.0)	≥15

Source: National Academy of Sciences.

yet discovered they are pregnant. Therefore, health organizations recommend that all prospective mothers follow a healthful diet based on the Food Guide Pyramid. That fact that about half the pregnancies in the United States are unplanned suggests that all women of child-bearing age who are capable of becoming pregnant should pay close attention to their food choices.

From the point of conception to the moment of birth, a normal pregnancy lasts about 40 weeks (9 months). For convenience, we often divide the time of pregnancy into **trimesters**, each lasting about 3 months. Pregnancy—also called **gestation**—begins when an egg, or ovum, is fertilized and becomes implanted in the wall of the uterus. It is here that the **placenta** forms, thus serving as the connecting organ between mother and fetus. The placenta contains a network of blood vessels from both mother and fetus that are in close proximity, allowing easy exchange of nutrients and other substances. The mother's nutritional health before conception is very important, because the uterus must be able to support the growth of the placenta in the first few days of pregnancy. The placenta also produces hormones needed to maintain pregnancy. If the placenta is poorly formed or if maternal support is compromised in any way, the fetus will fail to thrive. The term **low birth weight** is used for infants weighing less then 5.5 pounds; babies born before 37 weeks of gestation are referred to as **preterm** or **premature**. Low birth weight infants have a significantly greater chance of dying during their first year of life than normal weight infants; therefore, low birth weight is widely used as an indicator of future health status.

A woman's body weight before and during pregnancy can influence the health of both mother and fetus. Whether overweight or underweight, all prospective mothers should strive to normalize their body weight before becoming pregnant. Starting off at an appropriate weight can help minimize problems during pregnancy and increase the chances of delivering a healthy baby. Maternal obesity can increase the risk of infection, gestational diabetes, pregnancy-induced hypertension, and neural tube defects (see below). Women who are underweight and fail to gain adequately during their pregnancy are more likely to deliver low birth weight babies. Therefore, the amount of weight gain during pregnancy should be closely monitored. Recognizing that women of all sizes become pregnant, the National Academy of Sciences has developed guidelines for weight gain (table 10.1) that are based on a woman's Body Mass Index (BMI) before pregnancy. Note that the recommended weight gain for a "normal weight" woman during the course of a full-term pregnancy is 25–35 pounds (11–16 kg). This works out to about 1 pound per week during the second and third trimesters as the size of the fetus increases considerably. An overweight woman would be expected to gain much less during pregnancy, while an underweight women could gain as much as 40 pounds and still remain within an acceptable range. Also note that the BMI ranges used by the National Academy of Sciences to define "Low," "Normal," "High," and "Obese" are slightly different than the ranges used in the Dietary Guidelines for Americans (see Chapter 8).

To support a growing fetus, pregnant women need to consume more essential nutrients and total energy than nonpregnant women. Although there is great variation among individual women, total energy consumption generally needs to increase by 300 kilocalories per day, and only during the second and third trimester when fetal growth is greatest. This doesn't seem like very much when

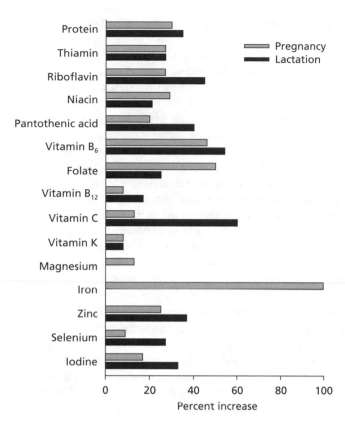

Figure 10.1 Percent increase in nutrient recommendations for pregnant and lactating women. The actual recommended amounts can be found in Appendix A. Values shown are based on the Dietary Reference Intakes (DRIs) for ages 19–30 or the Recommended Dietary Allowance (RDA) for ages 19–24.

you consider that 300 kilocalories is in two glasses of milk. But it's enough extra energy to provide 56,000 kilocalories over two trimesters.

A growing fetus also increases the demand for protein, vitamins, and minerals. Figure 10.1 shows how much the dietary recommendations increase for pregnant women above those for non-pregnant women aged 19–30 years. Extra protein is needed to build new tissues in the growing fetus as well as in the placenta, uterus, and breasts. Most adults living in the United States already consume double the dietary recommendation for protein, so the increased protein needs of pregnant women are easily met. The dietary recommendation for folate (or folic acid) increases 50% during pregnancy. Folate is involved in DNA synthesis and greater amounts are needed to keep up with the rapid cell division that occurs as the fetus develops. This is particularly important during the first few weeks of gestation when the brain and spinal cord are beginning to take shape. Inadequate amounts of folate will interrupt their formation, resulting in abnormalities called **neural tube defects**. One of the most common neural tube defects is **spina bifida**, in which the unprotected spinal cord protrudes out of the spinal column, causing varying degrees of paralysis and even death. The dietary recommendation for iron increases 100% during pregnancy, more than any other essential nutrient. This is because of the increased demand for red blood cells in both the mother and the growing fetus. A woman's blood volume significantly increases during pregnancy in order to handle the increased duties of nutrient and oxygen transport. Iron deficiency anemia is a common problem during pregnancy because doubling your intake of iron as recommended is difficult to achieve through diet alone. To prevent iron and folate deficiencies, some health care professionals recommend taking supplements. However it's also important to recognize that dietary supplements are not a substitute for a healthful diet that follows the Food Guide Pyramid. Women who are pregnant or planning on becoming pregnant should check with their physician, registered dietitian, or other qualified professional before taking supplements.

Pregnant women should be cautious about ingesting any substance in excess or those that have known effects on the developing fetus. Many drugs—whether illicit, prescription, or over-the-counter—have the potential to cause birth defects. Taking excessive amounts of vitamin A (and, to a lesser extent, vitamin D) can be toxic because it accumulates in the liver and other fatty tissues in both the mother and fetus. A single megadose of vitamin A can cause birth defects. Women who plan on taking a vitamin supplement during pregnancy should be aware that vitamin A supplementation is generally not advised during the first trimester, nor should the daily intake in the second or third trimester exceed the recommended amount of 800 µg (retinol equivalents), including dietary sources. Commercially available herbal supplements and herbal teas should be completely avoided during pregnancy because of their unknown composition and lack of information regarding their effects on a developing fetus. Although a consensus on caffeine has not yet been reached, many experts advise abstaining from caffeine as well. Alcohol consumption during pregnancy can also cause birth defects. **Fetal alcohol syndrome** refers to a host of abnormalities, including brain damage, altered facial features, and impaired vision. The critical levels at which these substances cause damage to the fetus are not well defined, so the best approach is to completely avoid them during pregnancy.

Another remarkable change that occurs during pregnancy is the preparation of breast tissue for **lactation**—the production and secretion of milk. Breasts enlarge as the milk-producing glands develop and as fat stores accumulates to ensure enough reserve energy to support lactation. The breasts are fully capable of producing milk by the start of the third trimester. After childbirth, the suckling of an infant causes the release of two hormones, **prolactin** and **oxytocin**, from the pituitary gland in the mother's brain. Prolactin stimulates milk production, whereas oxytocin causes the milk to move from its storage lobes to the nipple in a process known as the **let-down reflex**. The amount of milk produced depends on how frequent the infant nurses; when the infant stops breast-feeding, the breasts eventually "dry up" and milk production ceases. The milk that is produced during the first few days after childbirth is called **colostrum**, and is higher in protein and immune factors than mature breast milk.

Breast milk is the ideal food for growing infants. While **infant formula** can meet nutrient needs, breast milk contains the perfect balance of fat, carbohydrate, protein, vitamins, and minerals that an infant needs to thrive. Formulas are based on cows' milk or soy protein with a mixture of vegetable oils, added sugars, vitamins, and minerals. The intent of formula manufacturers is to mimic nature, but the proportion of nutrients in formulas is not exactly the same as breast milk. For example, breast milk contains two fatty acids (arachidonic acid and docohexaenoic acid) that are critical for normal growth, eyesight, and brain development. Most infant formulas do not contain these fatty acids, so an infant must make these in their cells from other fatty acids present in the formula. There is currently much debate in the scientific community about whether arachidonic acid and docohexaenoic acid should be included in infant formulas. Breast milk also contains digestive enzymes, hormones, growth factors, antibodies, and several other beneficial substances that are not present in infant formulas. Although formula feeding may be the only alternative in some cases, breast-feeding offers several benefits to both the infant and mother. Breast-feeding stimulates the uterus to return to normal size and helps to control postpartum bleeding. Breast-feeding is also convenient and inexpensive, it encourages bonding between mother and child, and it may reduce a woman's risk for osteoporosis, ovarian cancer, and breast cancer.

Women who breast-feed continue to provide all of the nutrients for their growing infant. Because the infant is more active and grows faster than the fetus, recommended intakes of several nutrients are greater during lactation than during pregnancy (figure 10.1). Nursing infants require on average about 700 kilocalories per day; therefore, the mother must provide this energy in addition to meeting her own energy needs. Since the mother's fat stores that accumulated during pregnancy can supply some of the energy, it is generally recommended that breast-feeding mothers consume a diet that provides about 500 kilocalories more than nonpregnant women. This recommendation assumes that the mother's diet will be sufficient to achieve and maintain a normal body weight throughout lactation while meeting the nutrient needs of her infant. Mothers who breast-feed must also consume plenty of fluids (about 8 cups per day) to encourage milk production and to prevent dehydration.

The chemical composition of breast milk is fairly constant, although it can be influenced by the mother's diet. Breast milk can take on some of the flavor and color characteristics of the mother's previous meal. First-time mothers are often concerned when their milk looks and smells unusual, but this is perfectly natural. In fact, studies have shown that infants prefer breast milk that is "flavored" with garlic, mint, vanilla, and other pleasantly odiferous foods consumed by the mother. On the down side, some substances—including alcohol—are distasteful to infants, so they tend to consume less. The color of breast milk is also influenced by the mother's diet. Green leafy vegetables such as spinach give breast milk a greenish tint; carrots and yellow vegetables impart a yellow color; and beets will turn breast milk a shade of pink. "Rusty pipe syndrome" is a brownish color in breast milk that can occur during the first few days of lactation and is due to trace amounts of blood from broken capillaries in the breast. This condition is harmless and disappears as the breast tissue adapts to lactation and breast-feeding.

Topic 10.2

From Infants to Teenagers

Key Points

Why is it so important to follow the growth pattern of children?
How effective are infant formulas at substituting for human milk?
In what ways can adult caregivers help establish healthful eating habits of children?

Some of the most dramatic changes in the human body occur between infancy and adulthood. The first year of life represents the most rapid rate of growth, in which infants *triple* their body weight. Increases in both height and body weight continue until about 18–20 years of age when adulthood is reached. An adequate and steady supply of nutrients is essential during the growing years because, unlike adults, children require nutrients to support the growth of new tissue in addition to supporting "routine" body functions. Although genetics influences the size of a person, diet and other environmental factors determine whether a person will attain their maximum potential size. Primary caregivers are key to establishing healthful eating habits that will help children achieve their full growth potential and promote good health throughout their lives.

An infant's **growth rate** is greater during the first few months than at any other time of life (figure 10.2). It's also during this time that an infant relies entirely on breast milk or liquid formula as the only source of nutrients. Providing a reliable commercial formula or making sure a nursing mother is receiving adequate nutrition is essential to optimizing an infant's growth. Growth curves similar to the ones shown in figure 10.2 are used by health care professionals to track the nutritional health of children. This type of chart is useful because the rate of growth may be more important

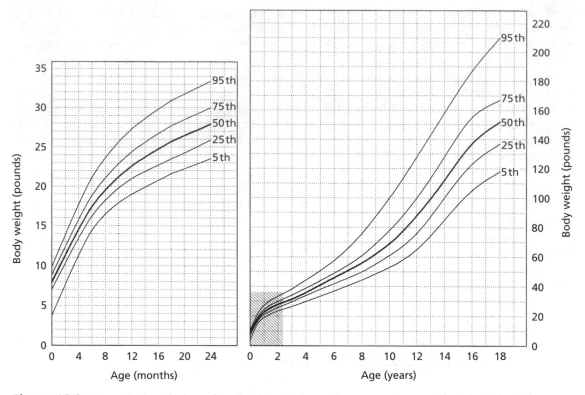

Figure 10.2 Growth chart for boys from birth to 18 years. The curves represent the 5th, 25th, 50th, 75th, and 95th percentile for boys living in the United States. Source: National Center for Health Statistics, Centers for Disease Control and Prevention.

than the absolute weight of a child. For example, a genetically small child may have a body weight that corresponds to the 5th percentile or below, but following the child's growth pattern will reveal whether he or she is being adequately fed. If an infant is receiving insufficient energy or if a nutrient deficiency develops, weight gain will begin to slow down or even decrease. Chronic nutrient deficiencies during childhood can cause irreversible impairments in growth and development that last into adulthood. The most severe impact of childhood malnutrition is on brain development, resulting in decreased cognitive function, poorer scholastic achievement, and long-term psychological and behavioral problems.

Human milk is perfectly designed to meet the nutritional needs of a growing infant, assuming the mother's nutritional status is adequate. Today's infant formulas are based on the composition of human milk and are generally well suited to substitute for breast-feeding. Federal regulations require that formula manufacturers comply with certain standards to ensure that nutritional needs are met. **Standard infant formulas** are made using diluted cows' milk, in which the fat is removed and replaced with vegetable oils. Also added are vitamins and minerals to match the proportion found in human milk. The primary carbohydrate in standard formulas, as in human milk, is lactose. It should be emphasized that while standard formulas are based on cows' milk, they are significantly modified to better meet the needs of a growing infant. Cows' milk should never be given directly to an infant because of its high protein content relative to human milk. The infant gastrointestinal tract is not fully developed and cannot handle the excessive amounts of protein. Furthermore, the type of protein found in cows' milk is different than the protein in

Table 10.2 Composition of milk and several infant formulas (per 100 kilocalories)

	Protein (g)	Fat (g)	Carbo-hydrate (g)	Iron (mg)	Calcium (mg)	Phosphorus (mg)
Human milk	1.5	6.0	9.3	0.05	45	19
Cows' milk (2% fat)	6.7	4.0	9.9	0.08	246	192
Cows' milk (skim)	9.3	0.5	14.0	0.08	352	288
Standard formulas (cows' milk-based)						
Enfamil	2.1	5.3	10.9	1.8	78	53
Gerber	2.2	5.4	10.7	1.8	76	57
Good Start	2.4	5.1	11.0	1.5	64	36
LactoFree	2.2	5.5	10.4	1.8	64	55
Similac	2.1	5.4	10.7	1.8	78	42
SMA	2.2	5.3	10.6	1.8	62	41
Soy protein-based formulas						
Alsoy	2.8	4.9	11.1	1.8	105	61
Isomil	2.7	5.5	10.1	1.8	105	75
Nursoy	2.7	5.3	10.2	1.8	89	62
Prosobee	3.0	5.3	10.0	1.8	105	83
Hydrolyzed protein formulas						
Alimentum	2.8	5.5	10.3	1.8	105	75
Nutramigen	2.8	5.0	11.0	1.9	94	63
Pregestimil	2.8	5.6	10.3	1.9	94	63

human milk and has a greater tendency to form hard curds in an infant's stomach. For this reason, **soy protein formulas** are available for infants who cannot tolerate the standard formulas. In addition, soy-based formulas are made with corn syrup and/or sucrose for infants who are lactose intolerant. For infants who are allergic to the protein found in both cows' milk and soy, a third type of formula is made with **hydrolyzed protein** in which the protein has been pre-digested. Regardless of which type of formula you choose, the American Academy of Pediatrics recommends that you select iron-fortified formulas because they better reflect the amount of iron provided in human milk.

A primary goal in the manufacturing of infant formulas is to mimic the levels of protein, fat, and carbohydrate in human milk (table 10.2). Cows' milk has significantly higher amounts of protein and certain minerals than human milk, therefore it must be diluted to reduce the concentration of protein so that it is closer to the protein concentration of human milk. One concern with standard formulas made with cows' milk is that the main protein (casein) is different than the protein found in human milk (lactalbumin) and tends to form hard curds in the infant gastrointestinal tract.

Solid foods can be introduced as soon as the infant is physical ready to receive them. This readiness depends on their ability to sit up, how well they can control head movement, and the development of their gastrointestinal tract. The American Academy of Pediatrics recommends that solid foods be introduced between the age of 4 and 6 months. Attempting to feed solid foods too early will be met with the **extrusion reflex** where the tongue is thrust forward, rejecting the spoon and its

Table 10.3 Foods to avoid during the first year

Foods to avoid	Explanation
Cows' milk	May cause allergic reaction; high protein content poorly tolerated; associated with iron deficiency
Egg whites	May cause allergic reaction
Peanuts and other nut products	May cause allergic reaction
Soy products	May cause allergic reaction
Wheat products	May cause allergic reaction
Fish and seafood	May cause allergic reaction
Honey and corn syrup	Contain bacteria spores causing botulism
Caffeinated foods and beverages	Unnecessarily stimulates the nervous system
Salted or spicy foods	Irritates the GI tract and stresses the kidneys
Sweetened juices and soft drinks	High sugar content promotes tooth decay; few nutritional benefits besides carbohydrate ("empty calories")
Foods that can cause choking	Hazardous foods include grapes, nuts, hot dogs, raw carrots, raisins, popcorn, chewing gum, apple pieces, hard candy, or any hard marble-size foods

contents. Although we use the term "solid foods," a baby's first foods should be pureed or liquefied and given only as a supplement to breast milk or formula. Gradually, the proportion of solid foods in an infant's diet can be increased so that by 1 year of age breast milk or formula is no longer necessary. Pureed foods of all type are available in the "baby food" section of the supermarket or they can be prepared at home using a blender, food processor, or baby food grinder. Rice cereal is often recommended as the first food because it is generally well tolerated, easily digested, and rarely causes allergic reactions. Table 10.3 lists certain foods that should be avoided during the first year because of their potential to cause harm.

Parents and other caregivers are directly responsible for shaping the **eating habits** of young children. Starting children out with good eating habits will increase their chances of a long and healthful life. Experts suggest that caregivers should offer a variety of food choices at mealtime, but let the toddler select which foods and how much they will eat. Toddlers have small stomachs and high energy needs, so they need to eat more frequently than the typical adult schedule of two or three large meals each day. Meals should be provided in a supportive environment where experimentation and exploration of food is encouraged. Food should never be given as a reward or denied as a punishment. Meals are a time for communication and building positive relations with our children. Teaching toddlers to feed themselves is an important stage of development that requires the caregiver to be patient and tolerant of messes. Children generally learn good table manners and healthful eating habits by watching adults, so it's important that caregivers model the type of behavior they wish their children to have.

The Food Guide Pyramid offers the best approach to creating nutritious and adequate meals for teenagers. Children of all ages should be provided with meals that offer variety from every food group represented on the Food Guide Pyramid. Of course, portion sizes will steadily increase as children get older. Many caregivers are often surprised at the shear volume of food that one teenage boy can consume in a day! Tremendous growth spurts usually occur between the onset of puberty (11–13 years of age) and young adulthood (figure 10.2). A child's body needs to grow, so it's important that a variety of nutritious foods are available throughout these critical years of development.

Topic 10.3

The Adult Years

> **Key Points**
>
> What factors contribute to longevity?
> What physiological changes occur with aging?
> How do these changes affect the nutritional status of older adults?

Humans are living longer than at any other time in history. During the past century, life expectancy in the United States has gained nearly 30 years and will likely rise in the future (figure 10.3). The increase in **life expectancy** in developed countries has been largely attributed to better infant health, prevention and treatment of diseases, and greater knowledge and application of nutrition. The twentieth century has seen many new discoveries—including the vitamins and other essential nutrients—that have profoundly influenced human life. The development of vaccines and medicinal drugs has also helped, but they would be of little use without an adequate diet. And while genetics does play a role in determining health, the genetic make-up of humans has not dramatically changed during the past century, indicating that a person's diet is truly the cornerstone of good health.

In contrast to the growing years in which new tissues are being made, an adult's diet is primarily used to maintain body functions. Consuming a "maintenance" diet that fulfills the body's needs while promoting good health should be a concern at every stage of adulthood. Many nutrition-related diseases take years to develop, suggesting that what we eat as young adults will influence our health later in life. Studies have shown that people who live longer are more likely to eat breakfast, more fruits and vegetables, and less saturated fat; they are also less likely to "diet;" and they have fewer fluctuations in body weight during their lifetime. Moreover, people who live longer tend to remain physically, mentally, and socially active throughout adulthood.

Progressing from young adult to middle-aged adult to older adult covers some 60 years on average and represents the process we call **aging**. Strictly speaking, aging is not something that

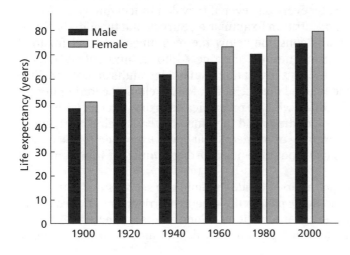

Figure 10.3 Life expectancy in the United States during the twentieth century. The most recent data available are from 1999. Source: National Center for Health Statistics, Centers for Disease Control and Prevention.

occurs only in the elderly; it begins at the earliest signs of life and continues until death. We don't usually refer to young children as aging ("growing" seems more acceptable), although aging is a time-dependent characteristic of all biological systems that is constantly moving forward. A few disreputable authors and product manufacturers have been promoting the notion that aging can be stopped or even reversed. From a biological point of view, this idea is utter nonsense. While it is possible to control certain "symptoms" of aging—such as wrinkled skin and gray hair—with cosmetic treatment, the underlying biological processes of aging are inescapable.

Aging is a normal consequence of life that results in many **physiological changes**. As people get older, these changes can have both direct and indirect impacts on nutritional status:

- Decreased muscle mass
- Decreased immune function
- Decreased organ function
- Decreased nutrient absorption
- Decreased hormone production
- Decreased taste, smell, and vision
- Decreased appetite
- Decreased mobility and flexibility
- Decreased thirst response
- Increased body fat
- Increased bone loss
- Dental problems

Aging is accompanied by a decline in human growth hormone, which normally stimulates skeletal and muscle growth. The result is decreased muscle mass and increased bone loss. Insulin production also declines with age, causing blood glucose levels to gradually increase. When coupled with increased body fat, this places older adults at risk for developing Type 2 diabetes mellitus. Organ function generally declines with age and can lead to impaired nutrient absorption, transport, and utilization in the body. Poor kidney function can cause water and electrolyte imbalance. Aging is also associated with delayed gastric emptying and a decline in the secretion of digestive juices. As immune function declines with age, susceptibility to infection and cancer increases.

Some physiological changes that occur with aging can affect nutritional status in indirect ways. Dental problems and a decline in the ability to taste and smell decrease the appeal and enjoyment of food, while limitations in mobility and vision make it difficult to shop for and prepare food. Diminished thirst response causes a decline in fluid intake, resulting in dehydration and constipation—common problems among older adults. To prevent dehydration, older adults need to consume the equivalent of 8 glasses of water every day even if they do not feel thirsty.

Recent data from the National Health and Nutrition Examination Survey and the Elderly Nutrition Program indicate that most older adults consume below the recommended level for total energy, folate, vitamin D, vitamin E, calcium, magnesium, and zinc. Although nutrient and energy requirements generally decrease with age, the data suggest that many older adults do not consume enough kilocalories to maintain body function and may be at risk for developing certain nutrient deficiencies. Of particular concern are individuals who are on medications that interact with nutrients in food. Some foods block the absorption of drugs and therefore decrease their effectiveness. Likewise, some drugs interfere with the absorption of nutrients that could lead to deficiencies. Patients should always check with their physician about the possible **drug–nutrient interactions** of the medications they are taking.

The Dietary Guidelines for Americans and the Food Guide Pyramid can serve as the foundation for a healthful diet, but special attention should be paid to the specific nutrients mentioned above and to possible drug–nutrient (and drug–drug) interactions. Older adults or their health care providers should select nutrient-dense foods when planning meals and may need to consider a vitamin and mineral supplement.

Application

Among the many factors in our environment that influence nutrition and health, television viewing is one of the most threatening to children. On average, children in the United States spend more time watching television than they do in school; two-thirds watch at least 2 hours of television per day. Television viewing can impact a child's nutritional status in several ways. First, time spent in front of the television decreases the opportunity for children to develop social, intellectual, and physical skills. Second, it encourages snacking behavior. The number of hours spent watching television correlates with the frequency of between-meal snacks. Third, it introduces children to foods they might not otherwise be exposed to. Television advertisers target children's programs for the promotion of snacks, desserts, beverages, and sweetened breakfast cereals. Consequently, children develop a preference for foods high in fat, sugar, and salt at an early age that will later influence their food choices as adults. Fourth, watching television requires no physical activity, except for the occasional trip to the kitchen. The incidence of childhood obesity has more than doubled in recent years, which experts have attributed to decreased physical activity. Studies have shown that children who watch at least 4 hours of television per day have more body fat and higher BMIs than children who watch 2 hours or less. Parents and other caregivers should limit the amount of time children spend watching television. The American Academy of Pediatrics recommends no more than 2 hours per day, although unplugging the television altogether doesn't seem like such a bad idea!

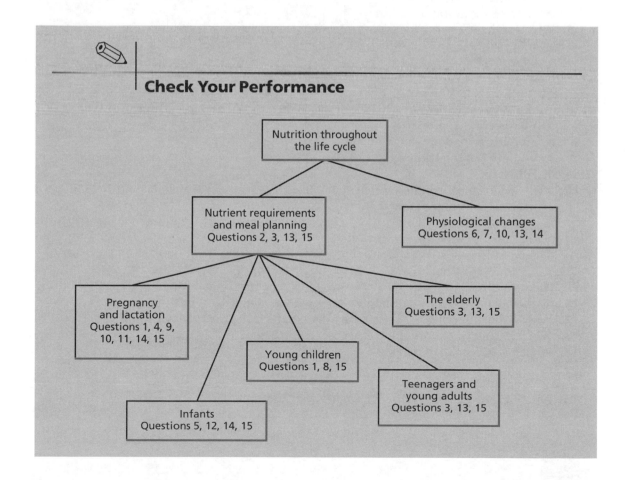

Check Your Performance

Nutrition throughout the life cycle

Nutrient requirements and meal planning
Questions 2, 3, 13, 15

Physiological changes
Questions 6, 7, 10, 13, 14

Pregnancy and lactation
Questions 1, 4, 9, 10, 11, 14, 15

The elderly
Questions 3, 13, 15

Young children
Questions 1, 8, 15

Teenagers and young adults
Questions 3, 13, 15

Infants
Questions 5, 12, 14, 15

Chapter Test

True/False
1. Being overweight before and during pregnancy is recommended because the excess body fat provides the energy reserves needed for the growing fetus
2. The best approach to feeding young children is to provide a variety of foods at mealtime, but let the child select what foods and how much he or she will eat
3. The Food Guide Pyramid, while useful for young adults, is not appropriate for people over 65 years of age
4. Consuming megadoses of vitamins during pregnancy can be toxic to the growing fetus
5. Solid foods should not be given to infants less than 1 year old

Multiple Choice
6. Life expectancy in the United States is currently
    a. 65–70 years
    b. 75–80 years
    c. 85–90 years
    d. 95–100 years
7. The clinical definition of "preterm" or "premature" refers to infants born before
    a. 37 weeks of gestation
    b. 38 weeks of gestation
    c. 39 weeks of gestation
    d. 40 weeks of gestation
8. Which of the following foods pose a choking hazard for young children?
    a. Grapes
    b. Popcorn
    c. Hot dogs
    d. All of the above
9. The recommended intakes of which nutrients increase the greatest during pregnancy?
    a. Vitamin A and vitamin D
    b. Protein and carbohydrate
    c. Vitamin E and selenium
    d. Folate and iron
10. What will happen if an infant is receiving insufficient amounts of dietary energy?
    a. Skin will become dry and scaly
    b. Hair will fall out
    c. Growth rate will slow down
    d. Bones will become fragile

Short Answer
11. List some of the dietary substances that should be avoided during pregnancy
12. What is the difference between standard infant formulas and soy-based formulas?
13. What lifestyle habits are associated with living longer?
14. What is the "let-down reflex"?

Essay
15. Describe how nutritional needs change at each stage of life

Further Reading

American Dietetic Association (1999) Position of the American Dietetic Association: nutrition standards for child-care programs. *Journal of the American Dietetic Association*, **99**, 981–8.

American Dietetic Association (2000) Position of the American Dietetic Association: nutrition, aging, and the continuum of care. *Journal of the American Dietetic Association*, **100**, 580–95.

Chen, C.C., Schilling, L.S. & Lyder, C.H. (2001) A concept analysis of malnutrition in the elderly. *Journal of Advanced Nursing*, **36**, 131–42.

Douglas, J. (1998) "Why won't my toddler eat"? *The Practitioner*, **242**, 516–22.

Floyd, R.L., Ebrahim, S.H., Boyle, C.A. & Gould, D.W. (1999) Observations from the CDC. Preventing alcohol-exposed pregnancies among women of childbearing age: the necessity of a preconceptional approach. *Journal of Women's Health & Gender-Based Medicine*, **8**, 733–6.

Freeland-Graves, J. & Nitzke, S. (2002) Position of the American Dietetic Association: total diet approach to communicating food and nutrition information. *Journal of the American Dietetic Association*, **102**, 100–8.

Guarderas, J.C. (2001) Is it food allergy? Differentiating the causes of adverse reactions to food. *Postgraduate Medicine*, **109**, 125–34.

Mangels, A.R. & Messina, V. (2001) Considerations in planning vegan diets: infants. *Journal of the American Dietetic Association*, **101**, 670–7.

Robinson, T.N. (2001) Television viewing and childhood obesity. *Pediatric Clinics of North America*, **48**, 1017–25.

Weaver, C.M., Proulx, W.R. & Heaney, R. (1999) Choices for achieving adequate dietary calcium with a vegetarian diet. *American Journal of Clinical Nutrition*, **70**(Suppl. 3), 543S–48S.

Part IV

Social and Economic Aspects of Nutrition

Chapter 11

Psychology of Nutrition

Many factors influence what, when, where, why, and how much we eat. In addition to the physical need to eat, there are several "external" factors that directly affect our food choices and eating habits. These external factors shape our attitudes and beliefs about food—what we like and don't like, what we find acceptable and unacceptable, what we think we should or shouldn't eat. This chapter examines many of the psychological aspects of nutrition and their importance in planning for and maintaining a healthful diet. The last section discusses abnormal eating behaviors and what can happen when these external influences become harmful.

Essential Background

❖ Appreciation of the cultural influences on human behavior
❖ Nutrient availability and dietary recommendations (Chapter 4)
❖ Influences on body composition (Chapter 8)

Topic 11.1

Food Choices

> **Key Points**
>
> What factors influence our food choices?
> Which factors are easily controlled and which ones are not?

Humans must eat to survive, yet food has much more meaning to us then merely survival. In many ways, the food we eat defines who we are as individuals and as a society. Celebrations and family gatherings are often centered around food. We sometimes select foods to project a desired image such as creativity, strength, or sensitivity. Food can provide comfort. Or we can use food as a sign of control by choosing certain foods or choosing not to eat. Religious practices, economics, cultural traditions, and geography also influence what we eat. Although the preference for certain foods may be genetically controlled, most of our food choices are influenced by our experiences and the environment in which we live. The following list shows many important factors that affect our food choices:

Personal influences
- Education
- Habits

- Perceived health beliefs
- Current health status
- Likes and dislikes

Cultural influences
- Customs and traditions
- Religious beliefs
- Acceptability
- Peer pressure
- Government policies

Practical influences
- Availability
- Convenience
- Cost
- School or occupation

Many of our **personal** food choices are shaped by early experiences. Parents and other primary care givers are directly responsible for the foods young children are exposed to and, therefore, can influence a child's likes and dislikes later in life. Many studies have shown that most adults choose foods because they taste good; but our personal preference of what tastes good is greatly influenced by the foods we consumed as children. Food preferences can also change as we learn more about foods and their influence on chronic diseases. For example, the growing belief that dietary fat increases the risk of coronary heart disease has caused Americans to consume more low-fat and no-fat foods during the past decade. An existing illness or physical condition may also determine a person's food selection. A person with osteoporosis, for example, may choose foods high in calcium and vitamin D, while a pregnant woman may increase her consumption of foods high in folate. And in some cases, a person may not be able to eat normally and, therefore, must be fed with nutrient solutions intravenously or through a stomach tube.

Our **cultural** environment has a strong influence on food choices. We are often unaware of our dietary traditions—such as eating eggs for breakfast—because we have become so accustomed to them. However, traditions in other cultures can seem very strange indeed. For example, grubs are considered dietary staples in many parts of Africa and South America, yet few people in North America would consider eating grubs. Peer pressure can strongly influence our food choices, particularly for young people who are eager to "fit in" with their group of friends. In many cultures, advertising can promote the consumption of single food products, but it can also influence overall eating patterns such as shifting to low-fat or high-fiber diets.

Religious beliefs also influence food choices. According to religious law, Jews may only eat foods that are deemed "kosher". *Kosher* is a Hebrew word meaning "fit" or "proper" and is given to foods that have been prepared according to traditional practices and specific standards. "Kosher certified" means that a rabbi trained in religious law and production methods has determined that the food was processed in accordance with these practices and standards. Contrary to popular belief, kosher foods are not merely blessed by the rabbi. Rather, the rabbi carefully inspects all ingredients, equipment, and methods of processing before the food can be certified as kosher. In some large-scale operations, food manufacturers pay a rabbi to be on the premises during the hours of production. Adhering to kosher practices is an important concern in the food industry, as the sale of kosher foods continues to increase and accounts for more than one-third of all packaged food products.

Several organizations in the United States offer kosher certification at the national and local levels. The Union of Orthodox Jewish Congregations of America certifies the majority of kosher products in the United States, and uses a circled "U" on food packaging to signify kosher. The Committee for the Furtherance of Torah Observations uses a circled "K" to signify kosher. Other certifying organizations use their own kosher symbols, which has led to some confusion.

Jewish law forbids the consumption of pork or pork-derived products. While the consumption of beef and lamb is acceptable, kosher meat must be hand-slaughtered by a specially trained rabbi. Jewish law also prohibits the consumption of meat and milk together. The word "parve" or "pareve" on food labels means that the product contains neither milk nor meat ingredients. Kosher foods that contain milk or milk-derived ingredients are indicated by a "D" following the main kosher symbol.

Similar to Jewish food practices, Muslims also adhere to certain food restrictions. "Halal" means "lawful" or "permitted," and many food manufacturers are now producing foods according to halal standards. Most foods are considered halal, with the important exception of pork and its byproducts, blood, and alcohol. Acceptable meat animals must be completely drained of blood during slaughter and the carcasses thoroughly washed. The restriction on alcohol means that vanilla extract and other flavorings in an alcohol carrier cannot be consumption. Other food additives derived from animals may also render the product "haram" or unacceptable. Halal foods are monitored by the Islamic Food and Nutrition Council of America, which designates halal on food labels using an "M" circled in a crescent.

Of the many **practical** issues affecting what people eat, food availability impacts more people worldwide than any other factor (see Chapter 4). Food choices in many parts of the world are limited to foods produced locally, whereas developed countries tend to enjoy a diverse food selection because of the ability to transport and store foods from distant locations. Even if foods are available, our lifestyles and economic status often affect what foods we choose to eat. More and more people are eating outside the home and relying on "fast food" for many of their meals. While this type of lifestyle is more expensive than preparing food at home, it is time-saving and convenient. Sometimes food choices are limited to school meal programs or what we are able to consume at our place of work. For people with limited incomes, foods are often made available through government and volunteer programs.

Although some people have limited access to food, most people who live in developed countries have the luxury of choosing just about any food they wish. In fact, the wide selection and accessibility of food makes it difficult for many people to stay in energy balance or to make specific dietary changes when needed. Assuming that a dietary change is warranted, studies have shown that small changes tend to be more long-lasting than drastic changes in diet. Small changes are less disruptive to a person's regular eating habits and are usually more manageable on a daily basis. In general, dietary changes are more successful when a person can continue to enjoy their favorite foods in moderation.

Topic 11.2

To Eat or Not to Eat

Key Points

What is the difference between hunger and appetite?
What is satiety?
How do hunger, satiety, and appetite affect our eating decisions?

The drive to eat is controlled by both physical and psychological urges. **Hunger** is our physical need for food and is controlled by internal body mechanisms. Hunger is associated with unpleasant sensations—headache, weakness, stomach pains, irritability—that occur when we haven't eaten for a while. Eating will cause the hunger sensations to disappear, suppressing our desire to continue eating. The opposite of hunger is **satiety**, which refers to the feeling of fullness and satisfaction that comes after food is consumed. As food is digested and absorbed, the internal mechanisms that control satiety are gradually reversed and hunger reappears.

The specific metabolic events that control hunger and satiety are not fully understood, although it is now widely believed that many factors are involved. Current research suggests that hunger and satiety are controlled through three major processes: (i) the presence or absence of food in the gastrointestinal tract; (ii) the level of nutrients in the blood; and (iii) the production of hormones and other chemical substances in the body. Most of these processes are thought to elicit their effects on hunger and satiety by affecting a part of the brain called the **hypothalamus**. Consuming food causes the stomach and small intestine to stretch, which sends nerve impulses to the hypothalamus, increasing satiety. Exposure of the hypothalamus to elevated concentrations of blood glucose, triglycerides, and amino acids—as would occur in the absorptive state—also promotes satiety. Furthermore, several hormones and hormone-like substance are known to influence both hunger and satiety by directly affecting the hypothalamus. While not completely understood, current research suggests that the events that cycle between hunger and satiety must stay in balance to prevent overeating. Obesity experts are concentrating their research efforts in this area in the hope of developing better treatment and prevention strategies for obesity.

In contrast to hunger, **appetite** is our psychological desire to eat. Appetite is triggered by external influences, such as the sight of a chocolate cheesecake or a juicy hamburger. Whereas hunger is an instinctive, protective mechanism that ensures survival, appetite is associated with the pleasurable aspects of eating and tends to guide our food choices. Being hungry can enhance a person's appetite, but having the desire to eat a certain food can occur even with a full stomach. In societies where the food supply is plentiful, food consumption is largely controlled by appetite, while hunger plays a secondary role. For example, we tend to eat according to the clock rather than hunger cues; we usually fill our plates regardless of how hungry we are; we avoid foods we dislike; and we often continue eating when our stomachs are full. Hunger sensations become more evident when we skip meals or during times of fasting.

Eating in response to appetite rather than hunger can lead to overeating. Consequently, being able to distinguish between hunger and appetite can help people who are trying to control their food intake and manage their body weight through dietary changes. The best way to start is to follow your body's natural cues. Wait until you are hungry before eating, then eat half the amount you are accustomed to. If you are still hungry, eat more—but only until the hunger sensations disappear. Studies have shown that people who eat with blindfolds eat less than normal (and less than they think they are eating). Learning to "listen" to your body is an effective way to stay in energy balance.

Several drugs and dietary supplements have been used to control appetite, although their effectiveness and safety is questionable. The most powerful drugs can only be obtained by prescription and should only be used under a doctor's supervision. Pondimin (fenfluramine) and Ionamin (phentermine) have been around for about 20 years and in more recent years were widely prescribed together in a popular combination known as Fen-Phen. Unfortunately, studies were never conducted and the Food and Drug Administration never approved of their use together. It was later found that the combination caused heart valve problems and was responsible for several deaths. Another prescription drug, Redux (dexfenluramine), was also linked to heart valve problems, so Pondimin and Redux were withdrawn from the market. Ionamin and another drug, Meridia (sibutramine), are still available with a doctor's prescription.

Nonprescription (over-the-counter) products used to suppress appetite include caffeine, fibers, benzocaine, and phenylpropanolamine. In addition to its ability to suppress appetite, caffeine is a diuretic and can give the impression of fat reduction by causing body water loss. Fibers can expand in the stomach by attracting water and thus give the filling of fullness. Excessive use of fibers increases the risk of dehydration. Benzocaine is an anesthetic and is applied to the tongue to deaden the taste buds, which is thought to reduce the desire to eat. Phenylpropanolamine is found in several over-the-counter appetite suppressants such as Dexatrim and is also the active ingredient in many cold remedies. Phenylpropanolamine should not be taken by people with diabetes, high blood pressure, or kidney or thyroid conditions.

Topic 11.3

Eating Disorders

> **Key Points**
>
> What is an eating disorder?
> What are the diagnostic criteria used to identify eating disorders?
> What factors contribute to the development of eating disorders?
> How are eating disorders treated?

Every society around the world has developed certain dietary patterns and attitudes about food that are considered "normal" by the majority of people living in those societies. For example, it is normal in some parts of the world to eat while sitting on the floor, to eat at certain times of the day, or to eat (or avoid) certain foods. Such eating behaviors evolve over time and are influenced by the many factors described earlier in this chapter. Within a given society, however, a person may develop eating behaviors or attitudes about food that deviate from the norm and would therefore be considered unusual or "abnormal." In the United States, we would generally consider it normal if a person reduced their fat intake, but it might be considered abnormal if a person tried to eliminate fat from their diet out of fear that dietary fat is toxic to the body. Abnormal eating behaviors can range from the seemingly harmless to extreme behaviors that result in bodily harm and even death. In all cases, these abnormal behaviors are driven by psychological disorders that are not fully understood by the medical community. When abnormal eating behaviors become harmful, the person is said to have an **eating disorder**. There are three main categories of eating disorders—anorexia nervosa, bulimia nervosa, and binge-eating disorder—although other types of abnormal eating behaviors have been described and are generally categorized as "eating disorders not otherwise specified." The following discussion will focus on the three main categories of eating disorders.

Anorexia nervosa is a severe eating disorder characterized by an intense fear of gaining weight. Individuals with anorexia nervosa develop a distorted view of their bodies, believing they are fat even when they are severely underweight. They are obsessed with food and constantly think about ways to avoid eating and to lose weight. Anorexia nervosa causes people to starve themselves or to engage in excessive exercise; they may also purge what little food they do consume by vomiting or by using laxatives. The effects of such behavior begin to show as muscle wasting, slowed mental function, slowed heart rate, dry lips and skin, and abnormal hair growth. In females, menstruation may become irregular and can completely stop. Clinicians use the following criteria to diagnosis anorexia nervosa:

- Refusal to maintain body weight at or above 85% of normal weight
- Intense fear of gaining weight or becoming fat, even though underweight
- Disturbed body image or denial of the seriousness of the low body weight
- Absence of at least three consecutive menstrual cycles

Anorexia nervosa is seen mainly in young Caucasian females of middle to upper class status, although it is becoming more common among males and other socioeconomic levels and ethnic groups. It is also seen among athletes who engage in weight-regulated activities such as wrestling and gymnastics. The vast majority of cases worldwide are found in affluent Western societies where being thin is encouraged and is often associated with success, beauty, and good health. Unfortunately, these values have been largely created by celebrity entertainers and magazine models whose thinness is unrealistic and unattainable for the majority of people. It should be no surprise that eating disorders are common throughout the entertainment industry. Nevertheless, the pressure placed on young people, particularly young females, to conform to society's expectations is a major contributor to the development of anorexia nervosa. Individuals with the condition tend to be perfectionists and seek to please others. Low self-esteem and the need for order and control in their lives (at least through food and exercise) are also major contributors.

The goal in treating anorexia nervosa is to resolve the psychological problems that cause the abnormal eating behavior. Treatment almost always requires counseling and, in severe cases, hospitalization, where food intake and exercise behaviors can be carefully monitored. Family therapy can be very helpful, particularly when parents or other family members are perceived by the patient as the source of the social pressures. Recovery also involves educating the patient about nutrition, meal planning, and healthy exercise habits. Only about half of the patients fully recover from anorexia nervosa—some deny their condition, while others have difficulty establishing rational thoughts about body weight. Seeking professional care at the first sign of trouble can increase the chances of recovery.

Individuals with **bulimia nervosa** are also preoccupied with body weight and body image, but unlike anorexia nervosa, they are drawn towards food rather than turning away from it. Bulimia nervosa is characterized by recurring episodes of massive overeating (called food **binges**), followed by **purging** to get rid of the excess food and kilocalories. Methods of purging may include forced vomiting and the use of laxatives, enemas, and diuretics. Binges are also followed by periods of fasting, dieting, and excessive exercise. Bulimics tend to eat in secret and may spend days planning their next bingeing and purging episode. The bingeing/purging/dieting cycle that develops can go unnoticed by friends and family for many years because bulimics are usually normal weight (or even overweight). The only outward signs of bulimia nervosa are caused by the frequent regurgitation of stomach acid, such as irritation of the throat and esophagus, swollen lips and jaw, mouth sores, and tooth decay. In contrast to anorexia nervosa, individuals with bulimia nervosa feel they have little or no control over food, particularly during a binge. Bulimia nervosa is diagnosed using the following criteria:

- Two or more binge-eating episodes per week for at least 3 months
- Purging or other inappropriate behavior to prevent weight gain
- Preoccupation with body weight and shape
- Feeling a lack of control over eating during bingeing

The causes of bulimia nervosa are not entirely clear, although depression and the feeling of disorder in one's life are frequently observed. Most bulimics are females who describe growing up in chaotic environments and feeling "lost in the shuffle." They tend to lack confidence and have low self-esteem. Like anorexia nervosa, treatment of bulimia nervosa focuses on identifying the psychological disturbances that led to the patients' abnormal behavior. Separating their eating habits from their emotions is critical during treatment and for the establishment of normal eating behavior. Even with nutritional and psychological therapy, many bulimics continue to deal with the urge to binge throughout their lives.

Health care professionals now recognize a third psychological condition called **binge-eating disorder**. It is characterized by recurrent episodes of binge eating in the absence of purging behavior. Individuals with binge-eating disorder are usually overweight and will consume several thousand kilocalories during a single binge. Unlike anorexia nervosa and bulimia nervosa, a large proportion of people with binge-eating disorder are male (about one-third). The following criteria are used to diagnose binge-eating disorder:

- Rapid consumption of extremely large amounts if food in a short period of time
- Two or more binge-eating episodes per week for at least 6 months
- Binge eating in isolation
- Feeling of lack of control over eating or inability to stop eating during a binge
- Feeling of self-hatred, guilt, depression, or disgust after a binge
- Absence of purging, fasting, or excessive exercise

As with other eating disorders, the treatment of binge-eating disorder focuses on the underlying psychological issues responsible for the abnormal behavior. Patients are often asked to keep a detailed food record, indicating what foods and how much they consumed during the day. More importantly, they must record their feelings, emotions, and other circumstances that prompted them to eat. The information is then used to develop alternative behaviors so that binge eating may be avoided in the future.

Women who participate in sports—particularly endurance sports and those that have body weight and appearance demands—have an increased incidence of eating disorders. Female athletes also have a much higher incidence of amenorrhea (lack of menses) than nonathletic women. Amenorrhea is associated with premature osteoporosis; consequently, amenorrheic athletes experience diminished bone density and an increased risk of bone fracture. The American College of Sports Medicine has given the name **Female Athlete Triad** to describe athletic women who have an eating disorder, amenorrhea, and decreased bone density. Treatment should include normalizing eating behaviors and estrogen replacement to restore menses and increase bone density. Oral contraceptives are often used for the purpose of estrogen replacement.

Understanding how eating disorders can be prevented in the first place offers the best strategy for a healthy future. Recognizing how society's expectations influence our eating habits is a good starting point. Knowing how hunger, satiety, and appetite all contribute to our food choices is also critical in establishing healthy eating habits.

Application

It's been a long day at school and Cheryl is finally back in her dorm room. Looking into the mirror, Cheryl feels disgusted with her 125-pound body. "Why can't I be thin and beautiful," she says to herself. But before starting yet another diet, Cheryl decides to plan one last binge. Her roommate is studying in the library tonight, so Cheryl walks down to the corner grocery store and buys a package of cookies, a large bag of potato chips, a quart of ice cream, and a dozen donuts before heading back to her room. She knows how pleasurable it will be bingeing on her favorite treats—but she also knows the guilt and self-hatred she will feel afterwards. Cheryl takes comfort in knowing that her guilt will later be flushed down the toilet along with the food. These emotions are very familiar to her.

No one sees Cheryl slip back into her room. She feels safe. Cheryl changes into her most comfortable jogging shorts and sweatshirt. It's 6:00 p.m. when Cheryl first opens the bag of potato chips. She crushes the chips into smaller pieces so she can eat them more quickly. Next come the cookies and donuts, which Cheryl likes to eat with alternating bites. She has saved the ice cream until last; it's 6:25 p.m. by the time she finishes the last spoonful. She has found that drinking warm water while she eats the ice cream helps prevent those cold headaches she used to get. Peeking outside her dorm room, Cheryl makes sure no one is in the bathroom before slipping into the stall. Alone and with her stomach bulging with pain, she rams her finger down her throat. This used to be the most difficult part for Cheryl, but she is surprised at how easy it has gotten over the years. In three massive heaves, Cheryl's ritual is nearly complete. She returns to her room, fixes her hair, and begins planning the diet she will start tomorrow . . .

Check Your Performance

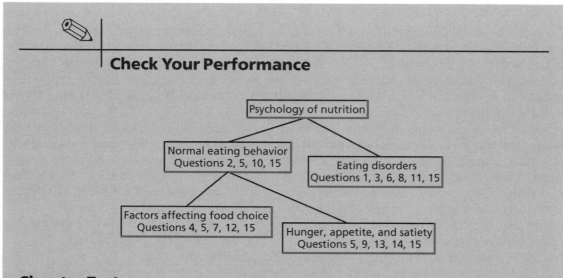

Chapter Test

True/False

1. The major cause of most eating disorders is a hormone imbalance
2. When trying to make long-term dietary changes, it's generally more successful to make drastic changes rather than small ones
3. People with bulimia nervosa can easily hide their disorder because the outward physical signs are not very obvious
4. Many of the food choices we make as adults are influenced by what we ate as children
5. Hunger is a strong influence on what foods we choose to eat

Multiple Choice

6. Successful treatment for eating disorders almost always includes
   a. Taking an introductory nutrition course
   b. Making an appointment with a registered dietitian
   c. Going on an energy-restrictive diet
   d. Psychological counseling

7. In economically developed countries, which of the following is unlikely to influence food choice?
   a. Taste
   b. Weather
   c. Religion
   d. Cost

8. What do all eating disorders have in common?
   a. They cause people to starve themselves
   b. They are characterized by overeating
   c. They are caused by psychological problems
   d. They are relatively harmless

9. Which of the following is associated with hunger?
   a. Physical need to eat
   b. Feeling full and satisfied
   c. Choosing your favorite food
   d. Having the desire to eat

10. The organ most responsible for regulating our eating habits is the
   a. Small intestine
   b. Stomach
   c. Liver
   d. Brain

Short Answer

11. What is an eating disorder?
12. Describe at least three practical influences that commonly affect food choice
13. How are hunger and appetite related to obesity?
14. What is satiety?

Essay

15. Describe the various ways in which society, friends, and family might contribute to eating disorders

Further Reading

American Dietetic Association (1994) Position of the American Dietetic Association: nutrition intervention in the treatment of anorexia nervosa, bulimia nervosa, and binge eating. *Journal of the American Dietetic Association*, **94**, 902–7.

Chapman, G.E., Melton, C.L. & Hammond, G.K. (1998) College and university students' breakfast consumption patterns: behaviours, beliefs, motivations and personal environmental influences. *Canadian Journal of Dietetic Practice and Research*, **59**, 176–82.

Dirks, R.T. & Duran, N. (2001) African-American dietary patterns at the beginning of the 20th century. *Journal of Nutrition*, **131**, 1881–9.

Duran, N. (2000) Dietary studies related to the United States diet prior to World War II: a bibliography for the study of changing American food habits over time. *Journal of Nutrition*, **130**, 1881–6.

Havel, P.J. (2001) Peripheral signals conveying metabolic information to the brain: short-term and long-term regulation of food intake and energy homeostasis. *Experimental Biology and Medicine (Maywood)*, **226**, 963–77.

Heber, D. & Bowerman, S. (2001) Applying science to changing dietary patterns. *Journal of Nutrition*, **131**(Suppl. 11), 3078S–81S.

Iraki, L., Bogdan, A., Hakkou, F., Amrani, N., Abkari, A. & Touitou, Y. (1997) Ramadan diet restrictions modify the circadian time structure in humans. A study on plasma gastrin, insulin, glucose, and calcium and on gastric pH. *Journal of Clinical Endocrinology and Metabolism*, **82**, 1261–73.

Nelson, M.S. & Jovanovic, L. (1987) Pregnancy, diabetes, and Jewish dietary law: the challenge for the pregnant diabetic woman who keeps kosher. *Journal of the American Dietetic Association*, **87**, 1054–7.

Schwartz, M.W. (2001) Brain pathways controlling food intake and body weight. *Experimental Biology and Medicine (Maywood)*, **226**, 978–81.

Siegel, M., Brisman, J. & Weinshel, M. (1997) *Surviving an Eating Disorder: Perspectives and Strategies for Family and Friends*. Gurze Books, Carlsbad, CA.

Slavin, J.L. (1999) Implementation of dietary modification. *American Journal of Medicine*, **106**(1A), 46S–9S.

Zizza, C., Siega-Riz, A.M. & Popkin, B.M. (2001) Significant increase in young adults' snacking between 1977–1978 and 1994–1996 represents a cause for concern! *Preventive Medicine*, **32**, 303–10.

Chapter 12

Use and Misuse of Nutrition Information

Nutrition information comes in many forms and from many sources. We are constantly bombarded with information about the purported benefits and hazards of things we eat. Some of what we read and hear is accurate, although a great deal of it is not. Advertisers might exaggerate the health benefits of a product in order to boost sales, while self-appointed consumer advocates are quick to denounce certain foods as being "bad" for health. Even scientists occasionally mislead the public by proclaiming their latest study as "definitive" when, in truth, no single study is so perfect in design that it provides the final word on health. An understanding of how nutrition information is generated and how it finds its way into our homes can help consumers judge its reliability. The first part of this chapter addresses the role of scientific research as the primary source of nutrition information and from which most health claims are made. Also discussed is the concept of disease risk and how it relates to human diets. The final section suggests ways of judging the reliability of nutrition information and how to recognize quackery and consumer fraud.

Essential Background

❖ Nutrient availability and dietary recommendations (Chapter 4)
❖ Factors affecting food choices (Chapter 11)
❖ Appreciation for the various ways news and information is delivered to consumers

Topic 12.1

From Research to Newspapers to Public Policy

> **Key Points**
>
> What is the scientific method?
> From what source do most consumers get their nutrition information?
> How are dietary recommendations for the general public formulated?

Most developed societies rely on **science** to explain nature. For many decades people have attempted to understand natural phenomena by using a systematic method of inquiry called the **scientific method**. This process has become the business of scientists, although being familiar with the scientific method can help consumers judge the reliability of nutrition information. The scientific method is really a "process of elimination" that slowly builds a picture of understanding one step at a time. In its purest form, the scientific method starts with an **observation** of something we would like to better understand. The next step is to propose a **hypothesis**—a statement that predicts one possible explanation for the observation. The hypothesis is then tested through **experimentation**. Finally, the results of the experiments are analyzed and a **conclusion** is made. The experiments should be designed so that the results will either support or refute the hypothesis. Seldom does an experiment address more than one hypothesis. Once a conclusion is made, another hypothesis may be proposed and the process started again.

Figure 12.1 illustrates how the scientific method can be applied to nutrition. Several years ago it was observed that a group of prisoners developed gastrointestinal disorders and an unexplained skin rash. The attending physician questioned whether the symptoms where caused by an infectious disease or whether they were related to the prisoners' diet. Based on his observation, the physician formulated two hypotheses that could be tested using experimentation. The first hypothesis was tested by studying whether the jailers who guarded the prisoners developed the same symptoms. After several weeks, it became clear that the jailers were not susceptible to the same disease, thus allowing the physician to conclude that the symptoms were not due to an infectious disease. The first hypothesis was then rejected. The second hypothesis was also tested through experimentation by replacing the prisoners' usual rice diet with a diet rich in fresh meats and vegetables. The symptoms began to disappear after a few days, thus providing the evidence needed to accept the second hypothesis.

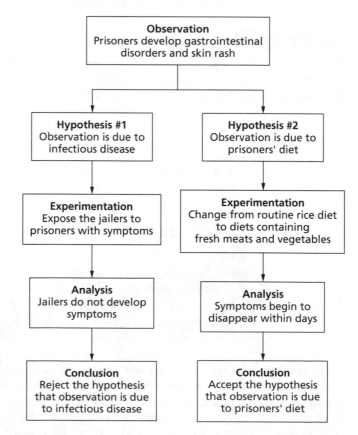

Figure 12.1 Illustration of the scientific method. Based on observations of natural events, the scientific method is a systematic approach to providing an explanation(s) for the observation. First, a hypothesis is proposed as a possible explanation. Second, an experiment is conducted to provide scientific evidence on which the hypothesis is either accepted or rejected. If rejected, more hypotheses are proposed and experiments conducted until consensus is reached regarding an explanation of the initial observation.

Although the physician made an important discovery, his results were far from definitive. Researchers were still left with many uncertainties regarding the prisoners' diet: Was the disease due to the presence of a harmful substance in the rice, or was the rice deficient in an essential nutrient that is found in meats and vegetables? And in any case, what might these substances be? To answer these questions, several more hypotheses and experiments followed over the next few years, eventually allowing researchers to conclude that the prisoners' disease (called pellagra) was due to a deficiency in the vitamin **niacin**. Using the scientific method, researchers were able to determine that the rice used in the prisoners' food was made with "polished" rice, in which the outer hull is removed from the rice kernel during processing. While niacin is naturally present in rice, it is found mostly in the outer hull. Substituting the rice diet with meats and vegetables—naturally good sources of niacin—eventually reversed the ill effects of niacin deficiency.

Using the scientific method to explain natural events and situations is analogous to putting together a very complicated jigsaw puzzle one piece at a time. Each time a hypothesis is tested with experimentation, one more piece of the puzzle is added. Clearly, this process is laborious and time-consuming, often taking many years or decades to understand a single observation. It is a continuous process that builds on previous knowledge, sometimes replacing outdated beliefs as the picture unfolds. Another example is the relationship between dietary cholesterol and serum cholesterol. It has long been believed that eating cholesterol-rich foods causes serum cholesterol to increase. But as more pieces of the cholesterol puzzle have been fitted together, it has become clear that dietary cholesterol has little impact on serum cholesterol levels in the vast majority of people.

At times the research business might seem like a game in which we try to guess the entire jigsaw puzzle with only a few scattered pieces in place. Although speculating about the implications of research studies is necessary in formulating further hypotheses, one should always keep in mind that single studies are merely individual puzzle pieces that, when viewed in isolation, can be misleading. First of all, there is no such thing as a perfect study. No matter how carefully designed and executed, there are always sources of error that creep into the experiments that must be accounted for. This is why most researchers used **statistics** to analyze their data. Statistics can quantify the experimental error in mathematical terms to help researchers judge the study's accuracy and reliability. Furthermore, individual studies—when conducted properly—should address only the hypothesis for which it was designed. Other intriguing questions will undoubtedly arise from each study, but in order to follow the scientific method, new hypotheses must be formulated and new experiments conducted. It's tempting to speculate about the broader significance of a single study, but doing so can leave false impressions that may not be supported by later studies.

Most consumers are unfamiliar with the scientific method and few people have the desire to read the professional journals in which research studies are published. Consequently, the public's major sources of nutrition information are popular sources such as newspapers, magazines, radio, television, and the internet. Reporting the results of studies through these popular means is an increasing and unfortunate trend. It's increasing because of the public's heightened awareness of diet and health issues, which makes nutrition research "newsworthy." It's unfortunate because without an understanding of the scientific method, consumers tend to place too much significance on the results of single studies, leading to frustration and confusion when contradictory stories appear in the news. In short, reporting the results of individual studies through these popular means serves no useful purpose and is largely to blame for the growing cynicism among consumers regarding scientific research.

The popular press is full of bogus and misleading nutrition information. A typical "women's" magazine will frequently have contradictory features touted on the cover: "Lose Weight Without Counting Calories" . . . "Desserts to Die For" . . . "Recipes That Lower Cholesterol." Moreover, the articles are often written by unqualified freelance writers who have no training or experience in the health field. Despite these obvious contradictions, many people get their nutrition information from sources that have little or no basis in fact. Keep in mind that the motive for publishing such information is almost always driven by monetary gain.

The usefulness of scientific research is best realized when the evidence is viewed in its entirety and **summarized** for the public's use. In other words, it is important to step back from the puzzle once in awhile and see what the picture looks like. The people involved in summarizing nutrition research are usually public health officials and other experts interested in diet and health relationships. Health organizations around the world, including many government agencies, frequently sponsor workshops and conferences in order to review the latest research on nutrition and other related topics. Two of the most comprehensive summary documents ever prepared were "The Surgeon General's Report on Nutrition and Health," published in 1988, and "Diet and Health: Implications for Reducing Chronic Disease Risk," published by the National Research Council in 1989. Both of these publications represent **public policy** documents on which many dietary recommendations are based.

Knowing how nutrition information is created and the various ways it is presented to the public can help consumers judge its usefulness and its limitations. As the larger picture of nutrition is slowly assembled through scientific research, it's important that individual studies are not misinterpreted as the final word on diet and health issues. Training ourselves to view nutrition information from a broader perspective requires effort. But by doing so, we are more likely to assess our own diets in their totality rather than singling out specific foods as either "good" or "bad." All foods can fit into a well-balanced diet.

Topic 12.2

Understanding Disease Risk

> ## Key Points
>
> How is disease risk calculated?
> What do "exposure" and "outcome" mean?
> What are the merits and limitations associated with disease risk calculations?

Webster's dictionary describes **risk** as "the chance of injury, damage, or loss." In nutrition, we use the term "risk" as a way of relating our diets with certain diseases or conditions. At first glance, this concept seems rather straightforward. However, closer examination reveals many uncertainties about what "risk" really means. We often read newspaper headlines such as, "High Fiber Diets Reduce the Risk of Colon Cancer," without questioning the meaning behind the headline. Does it mean that an individual can prevent colon cancer by consuming a high fiber diet? Does it mean that consuming dietary fiber will slow down cancer growth or lessen its severity? Does it mean that dietary fiber will improve health or extend life? Furthermore, is one type of fiber more effective than another? How much fiber should a person consume each day? And, finally, how does a person really know if increasing fiber intake affects whether he or she will get cancer later in life? These questions illustrate the ambiguity associated with the risk concept and how its casual use in the media is potentially misleading. In order for the concept of risk to have any practical application to nutrition and health, one must understand the limitations of the information it provides. Learning how disease risk is determined can help in this process.

Measuring disease risk requires two things—the ability to accurately measure what people eat, and the ability to document what diseases people develop. Once these measurements are made, then the relationship between them can be calculated mathematically and expressed in terms of risk. The numerous ways in which these data are collected make up a branch of science called **epidemiology**. The term **exposure** is used by epidemiologists to describe what people eat, while **outcome** is used to describe the occurrence and distribution of disease among populations. In our headline above, the relationship between dietary fiber and colon cancer was likely determined by first asking a group of study participants what they eat, and then following their progress for several years to see how many cases of colon cancer developed among them.

Many different tools are used to measure food intake (exposure), although the most popular are the 24-hour recall, the food record, and the food frequency questionnaire. The **24-hour recall** requires subjects to recall what foods and in what quantities they consumed during the past 24 hours. Other time periods may be used, but it is often difficult to remember what was consumed beyond 24 hours. The **food record**—sometimes called food diary—is perhaps more useful because it requires subjects to record the type and quantity of foods they consume at the time they are eating. Food records are usually kept for several days, which probably reflects a more accurate picture of overall dietary trends than a 24-hour recall. Both the 24-hour recall and food record require subjects to accurately assess the quantity of food consumed. Because most people have no previous experience in estimating portion size, epidemiologists must first train the study participants in how to determine food quantity. **Food frequency questionnaires** have gained in popularity in recent years because of their relatively low cost and simple administration. With this method, subjects are given a list of foods commonly consumed in the population and are asked to indicate how frequently those foods are consumed in their overall diet (figure 12.2). The advantage of food frequency questionnaires is that subjects only need to recognize what foods they have consumed on previous occasions. But unlike the 24-hour recall and food record methods, which document exactly what foods are consumed, food frequency methods are limited to only those foods that appear on the questionnaire. Validating the precision and accuracy of food frequency questionnaires has proven to be a difficult task. To quote epidemiologist Michael Nelson, "The history of nutritional epidemiology is littered with the skeletons of discarded questionnaires."

Just as dietary exposure can be assessed in different ways, several methods of quantifying disease outcomes are available, including disease incidence and disease prevalence. **Incidence** is the occurrence of an "event," usually the first clinical sign of a disease that appears over a specified period of time. Because incidence of disease is a function of time, it is most often called **incidence rate**. Calculation of an incidence rate involves selecting a suitable time interval and a population of interest that is free from disease at the beginning of the study. In the case of the colon cancer example, this would have required selecting subjects free of all clinical signs of the disease and then following the subjects for several years to determine how many new cases of colon cancer (fatal and nonfatal) developed during the study. By contrast, **prevalence** is the proportion or percentage of a population affected by the disease at a specific moment—a snapshot of a population at a single point in time. Prevalence does not consider the development of disease over time and is therefore not a rate. Prevalence includes both newly diagnosed cases and long-term survivors of disease, but its major shortcoming is that it does not account for people who have died from the disease.

Calculating disease risk is really a mathematical exercise in statistics. It is similar to flipping a coin and calculating the chance of getting "heads." In order to make this simple calculation, one must flip a coin many times—the more times you flip the coin, the more accurate your calculation will be. Similarly, epidemiologists must collect data from large **groups** of people to make disease risk calculations. The hope is that the results will reflect the entire population of people from which the study group was drawn. Obviously, there is no way to really know whether the study results can be applied to the whole population, since only a small portion of the population was studied. And

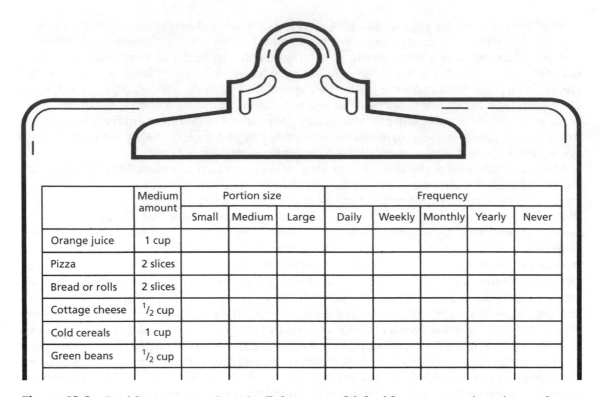

	Medium amount	Portion size			Frequency				
		Small	Medium	Large	Daily	Weekly	Monthly	Yearly	Never
Orange juice	1 cup								
Pizza	2 slices								
Bread or rolls	2 slices								
Cottage cheese	$^1/_2$ cup								
Cold cereals	1 cup								
Green beans	$^1/_2$ cup								

Figure 12.2 Food frequency questionnaire. To be most useful, food frequency questionnaires need to provide a list of foods that are relevant to the population being tested. They should also allow the respondent to choose portion size in addition to frequency of intake.

because disease risk calculations are made from "group data," it is impossible to know which **individuals** in the population will be affected by their diet and which ones will not. In other words, how do we know which individuals will benefit from increasing their fiber intake? Unfortunately, disease risk calculations are not designed to provide us with the answer, just as no one can know with absolute certainty whether a single flip of the coin will result in "heads."

Another shortcoming of disease risk calculations is that they cannot tell us if a direct cause-and-effect relationship exists between the exposure and the outcome—they can only tell us whether the exposure and outcome are **associated**. To illustrate the point, consider the fact that golfers have an increased risk of being struck by lightning. However, golfing does not *cause* lightning to strike, nor does a lightning storm *cause* someone to play golf. Neither lightning nor golfing are dependent on each other for either event to occur. No matter how carefully designed and executed, no nutritional epidemiologic study can demonstrate direct cause-and-effect relationships.

Nevertheless, there is still some merit to calculating disease risk. Epidemiologic studies form the basis for dietary recommendations, and even though disease risk numbers change somewhat with each new study, their collective information, when viewed from a broad perspective, can suggest which dietary trends are associated with good health and which ones are not. Disease risk calculations were never intended to address the specific health concerns of individuals, but rather to serve as a guidepost for whole populations. Furthermore, no single disease risk calculation should be viewed as definitive, nor should an apparent "new discovery" between diet and some disease be cause for alarm. Instead, the concept of disease risk is most useful when viewed as a tool for public health experts in making dietary recommendations for large numbers of people.

Topic 12.3

Interpreting Nutrition Information

> ### Key Points
>
> In what forms is nutrition information presented to the public?
> To what extent is the accuracy and reliability of nutrition information regulated?
> What questions should we ask ourselves when evaluating nutrition information?

Think of all the ways in which nutrition information finds its way into our lives: newspaper headlines, magazine articles, food labels, government reports, the internet, advertisements, infomercials, friends and family members. Most people want reliable nutrition information they can trust—information that will help them lead healthier lives. But with so much information available to consumers, it is often difficult to know what is accurate and what is not. Moreover, the nutrition information available to the public is not subject to any standard of truth and therefore can be offered as truth by virtually anyone, regardless of their nutrition background and experience. The ease with which nutrition information can be created and distributed, coupled with consumers' search for good health, has allowed fraudulent businesses and consumer scams to thrive. The marketplace is filled with bogus dietary plans and useless products that take advantage of vulnerable and unsuspecting consumers. Unfortunately, nutrition quackery not only robs people of their money, but can also rob them of their health. Every year there are reports of illness and death caused by hazardous products and unhealthy dietary plans. Learning how to question the reliability of nutrition information can help in sorting through the morass of products and unsubstantiated health claims:

Does someone stand to profit? Recognizing the motives behind nutrition information is one of the most revealing things we can do assess the reliability of the information. For example, on the one hand, government agencies and nonprofit health organizations provide nutrition information as a way of improving and maintaining the health of citizens. Their information is mainly based on scientific research and expert opinion, which has gone through multiple levels of evaluation and scrutiny. It sometimes takes years before the information is considered suitable for release to the general public. On the other hand, newspaper headlines and television news reports are meant to quickly capture your attention, sometimes at the expense of accuracy. Don't forget that a primary goal of newspapers, magazines, and television newscasts is to make money by amassing the largest number of readers and viewers possible. But the nutrition information that warrants our highest level of skepticism is the health claims made in advertising. When the sole motive is financial gain, the chance of fraudulent claims greatly increases, even when apparent experts are making the sales pitch.

Does the claim sound too good to be true? Then it probably is. The strategy of many fraudulent advertisements is to make unconventional and outrageous claims. Examples included such statements as "build muscle while you sleep," "stop aging now," and even "turn ugly fat into water, and flow it right out of your body by the gallon!" While the latter event would likely cause significant embarrassment if true, all of these statements basically defy logic. Yet, for some reason, we are drawn to them, perhaps in the same way we are drawn to tabloid newspapers to learn the latest "truth" about celebrities. We somehow know that the claims are not true, but we are still willing to spend money on bogus products in the hope that they just might work. Listen to your inner voice—trust your instincts—and resist the temptation of "buying in" to such wild claims.

Does the claim offer a simple solution to a complex problem? It's appealing to think that poor health can be magically improved by simply taking a dietary supplement. However, conditions such as obesity, arthritis, weak immunity, and the development of chronic diseases are terribly complex and still not fully understood by the medical community. Advertisers often take advantage of our limited knowledge by offering simple remedies that seem plausible on the surface and, more importantly, appeal to our personal concerns and suffering. But when one considers all of the genetic and environmental factors that contribute to poor health, the suggestion that a pill or an overnight diet plan will produce spontaneous improvements in health seems rather silly.

Are attractive terms used? Terms such as "breakthrough," "secret," "newly discovered," and "miraculous," are advertising ploys meant to capture your attention. But when compared to the laborious and methodical nature of scientific research, these terms have little meaning. Even the most important discoveries in nutrition have, in hindsight, required further research to establish their importance. In addition, descriptive terms such as "melts fat away," "speeds metabolism," "detoxifies," "boosts immune system," and "restores energy," are used by deceptive advertisers to tell us what the product or dietary plan is supposed to do. The latter expressions can sound convincing, especially when scientific words are used. However, such nonsense terms have no basis in medical science.

Are testimonials or expert endorsements used? Personal testimony can be very convincing—in fact, our judicial system is founded on personal testimony. The problem is that the use of testimonials in promoting nutrition information requires no verification. And assuming documentation is available, it's practically impossible to validate. Before-and-after photographs are frequently used in conjunction with testimonials—it seems even more convincing when we see the person who is providing the testimony. Particularly deceitful are advertisements that use so-called experts to provide the nutrition information. Consumers are more likely to buy something if it is endorsed by someone with MD or PhD following their name. Regardless of their credentials, you can be certain that these "experts" are being paid for their endorsement or they have a financial interest in the product or service being sold.

Are studies cited? As mentioned earlier in this chapter, reliable nutrition information is built on scientific research. Every study conducted provides a small piece of information that is used to slowly build a larger picture of understanding. In this context, we should never assume to have the definitive answer about diet and health issues based on the results of one study. Yet many advertisements, newspaper headlines, and television news reports will offer the results of single studies as "proof" that we finally know the solution to a troublesome health problem. Moreover, some advertisements claim to have research proof when, in fact, no research data exist. If the nutrition information is truly based on scientific research, then the studies should be available at most university and medical school libraries or accessed through the reference desk at most public libraries. Information about authentic studies is almost never provided in advertisements.

Is there reference to an exotic place? Distributors of disreputable nutrition information want you to believe that the best products and dietary plans come from places other than where you live. It's common to see statements such as, "Made from our special Swedish formula," or "Imported from the rainforests of Brazil," or "Now available in America after overwhelming success in Europe." Market tests have shown that the more exotic the location sounds, the more money consumers are willing to pay.

Because there are few laws regulating the nature of nutrition information or how it is made available to the public, we must adopt our own personal system of evaluating its accuracy and

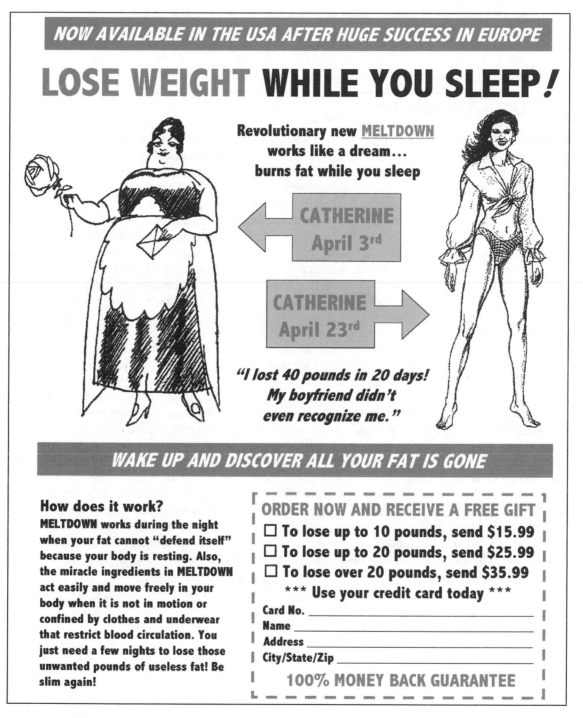

Figure 12.3 Typical weight-loss advertisement. How many "red flags" can you find in this advertisement that indicate it is fraudulent?

reliability. In figure 12.3, how many "red flags" can you find that indicate the advertisement is fraudulent?

Application

More and more people are turning to the internet for nutrition information. Consequently, several government agencies and nonprofit health organizations have created websites to provide consumers with reliable information. Among the most useful government websites related to nutrition are the US Department of Agriculture (www.usda.gov), the US Department of Health and Human Services (www.os.dhhs.gov), and the Centers for Disease Control and Prevention (www.cdc.gov). In addition, several nonprofit and volunteer organizations have been established that provide current and accurate information on their websites. Most of these organizations are managed by scientists and professionals in the area of food, nutrition, and health, and they include the American Dietetic Association (www.eatright.org), the American Medical Association (www.ama-assn.org), the International Food Information Council (www.ific.org), and the International Life Sciences Institute (www.ilsi.org). Some organizations have been created to provide information on specific nutrition-related disorders, including the American Cancer Society (www.cancer.org), the American Diabetes Association (www.diabetes.org), the American Heart Association (www.americanheart.org), and the National Osteoporosis Foundation (www.nof.org). While this is not an exhaustive list, all of these organizations strive to publish the most reliable and up-to-date information for the general public. Their common goal is to promote good health by highlighting dietary habits associated with longevity and increased quality of life. In contrast to these trustworthy organizations, consumers should be wary of organizations and websites whose only mission, it seems, is to condemn certain foods. In recent years, one consumer organization has been particularly aggressive in condemning foods by placing theater popcorn, deli sandwiches, and Italian, Mexican and Chinese food all at the top of their hit list. However, just as no single food produces magical health benefits, eating a serving of fettuccini alfredo once in a while will not cause an instant heart attack. Suggesting that certain foods are uniquely hazardous creates undue fear and shifts attention away from the importance of planning an overall healthful diet that focuses on variety, balance, and moderation. When searching for information on the internet, be cautious of organizations and websites that condemn or promote single food items, those that charge an access fee, and those that are not linked to other reputable sources of nutrition information.

Check Your Performance

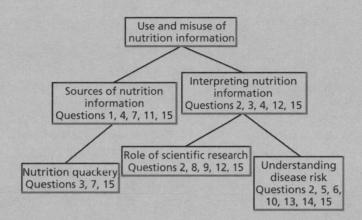

Chapter Test

True/False

1. One of the best sources of reliable nutrition information is the Surgeon General's Report on Nutrition and Health

2. The "food record" is the only method of assessing what people eat that does not require information on portion size

3. The use of testimonials in advertising is a sure indicator that the advertisement is promoting reliable nutrition information

4. All foods can fit into a healthful diet built on variety, balance, and moderation

5. Disease risk calculations can positively identify individuals within a population who will develop chronic diseases

Multiple Choice

6. The biggest disadvantage of using "prevalence" to document disease outcomes is
    a. It relies on self-reporting by the study participants
    b. It can only be used for male subjects
    c. It does not include fatal cases of disease
    d. It excludes people under 30 years of age

7. Which of the following newspaper headlines is most likely to represent reliable nutrition information?
    a. "Daily dose of vitamin D dramatically decreases diabetes"
    b. "Long-term study shows yellow squash reduces risk of heart disease"
    c. "Pink grapefruit can lower your risk of colon cancer"
    d. "Latest government report shows Americans are consuming more calories"

8. The scientific method can be summarized in the following sequence
    a. Proposition → experimentation → conclusion → observation
    b. Observation → hypothesis → experimentation → conclusion
    c. Experimentation → hypothesis → conclusion → publication
    d. Supposition → experimentation → hypothesis → conclusion

9. The study between diet and disease relationships in humans is called
   a. Epidemiology
   b. Nutripathy
   c. Ingestology
   d. Consumology

10. Why has the use of food frequency questionnaires by nutrition researchers increased in recent years?
   a. They are relatively simple to administer
   b. They require no prior training of study participants
   c. They are relatively inexpensive
   d. All of the above

Short Answer

11. Why are the Dietary Guidelines for Americans considered a reliable source of nutrition and health information?
12. In what ways is scientific research like assembling a jigsaw puzzle?
13. In epidemiology, what does it mean when an exposure and an outcome are "associated"?
14. What is a hypothesis?

Essay

15. Describe how you would judge the accuracy and reliability of the information in a newspaper article that had the headline, "High Fat Diets Increase Risk of Breast Cancer"

Further Reading

Anderson, J.G. (2000) Health information on the Internet: let the viewer beware (caveat viewor). *MD Computing*, **17**, 19–21.

Ashley, J.M. & Jarvis, W.T. (1995) Position of the American Dietetic Association: food and nutrition misinformation. *Journal of the American Dietetic Association*, **95**, 705–7.

Barrett, S. (1997) Quackwatch: Your Guide to Health Fraud, Quackery, and Intelligent Decisions. (http://www.quackwatch.com/) Accessed 13 Jan 2002.

Freeland-Graves, J. & Nitzke, S. (2002) Position of the American Dietetic Association: total diet approach to communicating food and nutrition information. *Journal of the American Dietetic Association*, **102**, 100–8.

Lee, R.D. & Nieman, D.C. (1996) *Nutritional Assessment*, 2nd ed. Mosby/McGraw-Hill, St Louis.

Massey, P.B. (2002) Dietary supplements. *Medical Clinics of North America*, **86**, 127–47.

Rodriquez, J.C. (1999) Legal, ethical, and professional issues to consider when communicating via the Internet: a suggest response model and policy. *Journal of the American Dietetic Association*, **99**, 1428–32.

Ross, J.F. (1999) *The Polar Bear Strategy: Reflections on Risk in Modern Life*. Perseus Books, Reading, MA.

Rowe, S. (2001) Communicating science-based food and nutrition information. *Journal of the American Dietetic Association*, **101**, 1145–6.

Short, S.H. (1994) Health quackery: our role as professionals. *Journal of the American Dietetic Association*, **94**, 607–11.

Chapter 13

The Food Industry

For generations, humans have grown, hunted, or gathered their food in order to survive. But with today's modern agricultural and technological advances, humans no longer need to rely on their own farming or hunting skills for survival. Food is now mass produced and widely distributed, so that people living in developed countries can spend their time on other activities. Supermarket shelves are stocked with fresh, frozen, canned, and packaged foods of all kinds and from every region of the world. We now depend on the **food industry** to provide us with a safe and wholesome food supply. Managing and coordinating such a large endeavor is the shared responsibility of food companies and government agencies to ensure certain standards of safety and quality.

Essential Background

❖ Major nutrient classes and their functions (Chapter 2)
❖ Nutrient availability and dietary recommendations (Chapter 4)
❖ Accessing and interpreting nutrition information (Chapter 12)

Topic 13.1

Food Technology

> **Key Points**
>
> What are the primary goals of the food processing industry?
> In what ways does food technology increase nutrient availability?
> What are the risks and benefits of using food additives?

Much of the food we consume has been prepared or handled in some way by industry. Advances in **food processing** technology have greatly improved the safety, wholesomeness, and enjoyment of foods. For example, pasteurizing (heating) milk destroys disease-causing bacteria commonly found in raw milk, thus making it safer to drink. At first glance, it may seem more "nutritious" to drink raw milk, but doing so greatly increases the risk of becoming ill. The modern techniques used in processing, packaging, and storing foods are also responsible for the wide variety and abundance of foods available to us. Without food processing, the health of entire populations would be compromised.

The two most fundamental goals of food processing are to minimize spoilage (increase a food's **shelf life**) and make food safer. To accomplish these goals, processing techniques are aimed at

Table 13.1 Common food additives and their function

Food additive	Function	Comments
Ascorbic acid (sodium ascorbate)	Preservative; nutrient	Inhibits oxidation and increases shelf life Ascorbic acid is another term for vitamin C
Baking soda (sodium bicarbonate)	Leavening agent	Creates small gas bubbles in baked goods, making them light and airy
Beet extract	Coloring agent	Provides red color
Beta-carotene	Preservative; coloring agent; nutrient	Inhibits oxidation and increases shelf life Provides yellow color Is a form of vitamin A
Carrageenan	Thickener; emulsifier	Helps thicken liquid foods Prevents fats and oils from separating from other liquid ingredients
Calcium silicate	Anti-caking agent	Keeps dry powdery foods free flowing
Folic acid	Nutrient	Essential nutrient added to grain products such as pasta and flour
Guar gum	Thickener	Helps thicken liquid foods Many other natural "gums" are used in the food industry
Lecithin	Emulsifier	Prevents fats and oils from separating from other liquid ingredients Found naturally in soybeans and corn
Monosodium glutamate (MSG)	Flavor enhancer	Often used in meats, sauces, and soups Is tasteless by itself
Pectin	Thickener	Used in making jams and jellies Considered a dietary fiber
Phosphoric acid	Increases acidity	Provides tartness to foods Used primarily in carbonated soft drinks
Salt	Preservative; flavor enhancer	Used extensively in the food industry to prevent growth of microorganisms Added to many savory foods
Sugar	Preservative; flavor enhancer; sweetener	Used extensively in the food industry to prevent growth of microorganisms Enhances flavor even in non-dessert foods
Tumeric extract	Coloring agent	Provides yellow color

preventing the growth of microorganisms that cause food spoilage or those that make you sick when consumed. Perhaps the most widely used method to inhibit the growth of microorganisms is the application of **high temperatures**. Cooking has been used for centuries to ensure food safety and still represents an important food processing technique in industry and in the home. **Pasteurization** (medium high temperature), **sterilization** (very high temperature), and **canning** methods all rely on high-temperature processing to kill microorganisms. Placing foods at **cold temperatures** also inhibits the growth of microorganisms and is an effective way to preserve food. The widespread use of home refrigerators and freezers has occurred only in the past few decades and has allowed the food industry to create a vast selection of the refrigerated and frozen food products that we enjoy today. Before modern kitchen appliances, however, people relied mainly on cooking as the primary way to preserve foods and to make them safe for consumption. Other traditional methods of preserving food are **fermentation**, **smoking**, and **drying**. Although these methods are somewhat obsolete compared to modern techniques of food preservation, they are still needed to make certain foods such as sauerkraut, pastrami, wine, smoked fish, raisins, and beef jerky.

Another way to preserve food is through the use of **food additives**. While the food industry is continually developing new food additives, the concept is not new. The addition of sugar and salt to foods to kill microorganisms and to extend the foods' shelf life has been used for centuries. Mixing sugar with fruit has long been known to preserve fruit and is the first step in making jams and jellies—sometimes called "preserves." Adding salt to meat and fish was common practice aboard sailing vessels and allowed these foods to be stored for several weeks or months without spoiling. It is interesting to note how early food processing techniques have influenced the taste preferences of modern societies. We have become accustomed to having sugar or salt in our food, and many people feel that their absence leaves food tasting bland and undesirable.

In the past century, food supplies have gradually shifted from family farms to grocery stores due to mass production and increased availability of foods, which has eliminated the need for people to grow their own food. As a result, consumers have steadily placed greater demands on the food industry for safe, long-lasting, high-quality foods at a reasonable price. To meet these demands, the food industry uses food additives that—in addition to preventing the growth of microorganisms—help protect and enhance color, flavor, and texture. Table 13.1 shows some common food additives and their functions that help to improve food quality.

A number of coloring agents are approved for food use in the United States. Some color additives require certification by the Food and Drug Administration (FDA), while others are exempt from certification. Tracing the history of food color in the United States reveals why regulation and certification became necessary.

Prior to the 1900s, a host of substances were added to foods not only to enhance their color, but also to disguise foods that were beginning to spoil. Many of these additives were later found to be quite poisonous, such as red lead, mercury sulfide, and copper arsenate. Moreover, textile dyes from coal tar often found their way into the food supply. In an attempt to impose some control, Congress passed The Food and Drug Act of 1906, which established a volunteer program for certification of synthetic color additives. The Food, Drug, and Cosmetic Act of 1938 instituted mandatory certification and required that each batch of colorant be chemically tested for impurities and to maintain consistency. The Color Additives Amendment of 1960 legally defined color additives and continued the mandatory certification of each color batch. More importantly, the amendment required that all color additives be tested for toxicity and cancer-causing potential before receiving approval. Because of the stringent testing procedures, many colorants have failed to "make the cut" and are no longer available for use in the United States. Currently, there are only seven colorants certified by the FDA for use in food and are designated "FD&C" colors in keeping with The Food, Drug, and Cosmetic Act of 1938:

- FD&C Yellow No. 5 (canary yellow)
- FD&C Yellow No. 6 (orange-yellow)
- FD&C Red No. 40 (fire engine red)
- FD&C Red No. 3 (watermelon red)
- FD&C Blue No. 2 (royal blue)
- FD&C Blue No. 1 (light blue)
- FD&C Green No. 3 (teal-green)

The Nutrition Labeling and Education Act of 1990 requires that FDA-certified color additives be listed individually on food labels (e.g., "FD&C Yellow No. 5" or simply "Yellow 5"). Certification requires that manufacturers submit a sample of each color batch to the FDA for chemical analysis. This ensures consistency and that every batch is chemically identical to the substance used in the toxicity studies upon which certification was originally granted.

Certified colors are available as FD&C dyes and FD&C lakes. Dyes are water soluble and exhibit their color by being dissolved. FD&C dyes are used in water-based foods such as beverages, gelatin mixes, ice cream, and jams and jellies. They are also used in processed foods made from water-based dough (such as breakfast cereals and snack foods). By contrast, lakes are insoluble pigments that color by dispersion. Lakes are made by chemically converting dyes into aluminum salts. FD&C lakes are used in a variety of foods where water-soluble dyes are not suitable. For example, striped candies have less color "bleed" if lakes are used. FD&C lakes are also used in chewing gum, cake mixes, icings, cream centers, and fruit fillings. Some foods—such as M&M's candies—use a combination of lakes and dyes. Food labels must indicate a lake by listing the name of the corresponding dye, following by the word "lake" (e.g., "FD&C Yellow No. 5—Aluminum Lake" or simply "Yellow 5 Lake").

Natural coloring agents—such as annatto extract, caramel, beta-carotene, carrot oil, paprika, and vegetable juices—are exempt from certification. Because natural color additives do not necessarily occur naturally in the foods to which they are added, they must be listed on food labels as an added ingredient. Their full name may be used or simply listed as "artificial color."

Other food additives are specifically intended to enhance the nutritional quality of food and therefore promote health. **Fortification** is the general term used to describe the addition of nutrients to food. Processing of food can sometimes result in nutrient losses. The term **enrichment** refers to a type of fortification in which nutrients are added to foods to replace those lost during processing. An example is the loss and subsequent replenishment of certain vitamins during the milling of wheat flour. Alternatively, some foods are fortified with nutrients that are not ordinarily present in the food. Examples of this are calcium-fortified orange juice and vitamin D-fortified milk. Food manufacturers are now taking this concept one step further by fortifying foods with nutrients and other natural substances believed to have therapeutic properties in promoting health. The term **functional food** is used to describe this relatively new approach to food product development (see Topic 13.4).

Many misconceptions about food additives have caused some consumers to view them as dangerous and unhealthy. Food additives used in the United States are strictly regulated by the Food and Drug Administration (FDA), and their safety is extensively tested before they can be used in the food supply. The notion that all food additives are "unnatural" chemicals created in the laboratory is somewhat misleading. Most food additives are actually substances found in nature and purified from natural sources. Carrageenan, for example, is a thickening agent that comes from seaweed that grows in the Atlantic Ocean. Nevertheless, some substances in food, whether they were intentionally added or are naturally present, are known to cause metabolic disturbances in some people. Nothing in the food supply is completely and absolutely devoid of risks—even water can become toxic if consumed in excess. Some people cannot consume monosodium glutamate (MSG) because it causes headache and flushing, yet others have no adverse reaction to MSG and rather enjoy the enhanced flavor of food that MSG provides. Whether we choose to consume foods containing additives should be a personal decision based on reliable information and what we believe is best for our own health and well being.

Topic 13.2

Food-Borne Illness

Key Points

What causes food-borne illness?
What is the difference between food-borne infection and food-borne intoxication?
How can food-borne illness be avoided?

The Centers for Disease Control and Prevention estimates that 3–10% of the population suffers from a **food-borne illness**. Consumption of contaminants in food and water can cause flu-like symptoms such as diarrhea, headache, nausea, and even death in severe cases. Many people who experience mild symptoms of food-borne illness don't even realize their discomfort is connected to something they ate. Because true influenza symptoms usually last several days, most cases of the "24-hour flu" are very likely food-borne illnesses. Treatment for food-borne illness includes drinking plenty of fluids, getting bed rest, washing hands frequently, and avoiding contact with food while diarrhea is present. Severe food-borne illness may require prompt medical attention.

Most food-borne illness in the United States is caused by eating food contaminated with micro-organisms called **pathogens**. Pathogenic microorganisms include bacteria, viruses, molds, and parasites (protozoa), but the majority of food-borne illness is caused by bacteria (table 13.2). Certain bacteria have the ability to grow in the gastrointestinal tract and spread to other tissue. This type of illness of called a **food-borne infection**. By contrast, some bacteria produce toxins in food or in the body, causing **food-borne intoxication**. Chemical toxins in the environment can also end up in the food supply, resulting in food-borne intoxication. It only takes a small amount of toxin to cause illness, whereas food-borne infection requires the ingestion of relatively large numbers of bacteria. Consequently, the harm caused by contaminants in food depends on the type and amount of pathogen and/or toxin, the length of time over which it is consumed, and the size and health status of the consumer.

The risk of food-borne illness can be decreased by proper food selection, preparation, and storage. Consumers should choose the freshest meats and produce, select frozen foods that have been kept at constant temperatures, and avoid packages with broken seals or contents that appear spoiled. Once at home, steps can be taken to minimize the introduction of pathogens during food preparation. Kitchen surfaces, hands and cooking utensils should be cleaned between each preparation step. **Cross-contamination**—the transfer of microorganisms from one food to another—commonly causes food-borne illness, especially when bacteria on raw animal products come in contact with foods that can support their growth. Thorough cooking of foods and the use of pasteurized products further help to reduce contamination. After food is prepared and cooked, never let it stand at room temperature for more than 1–2 hours—refrigerate or freeze as soon as possible. When reheating food, make sure the temperature reaches at least 165°F so that pathogens are destroyed. In general, treat all foods as potential sources of food-borne illness. When in doubt, throw it out!

In addition to the role consumers play in limiting the risks of developing food-borne illness, the food supply is monitored for safety by food manufacturers and regulatory agencies at the local, state, federal, and international levels. In the United States a system to improve food safety during processing and manufacturing has been developed called **Hazard Analysis Critical Control Point** (HACCP). Using HACCP principles offers a way of preventing food contamination, monitoring food processing methods, and tracking contaminated foods to prevent food-borne illness. Each processor and manufacturer is required to set up their own HACCP plan so that critical steps in the food handling process can be identified.

Contaminants such as pesticide residue and industrial wastes that leach into the environment can find their way into the food supply. In addition, some foods contain **natural toxins** such as goitrogens in cabbage, cyanogens in lima beans, and solanine in green potatoes. In general, the trace amounts of toxins in and on food products pose little risk to humans. Nevertheless, some people choose to avoid potential toxins altogether by selecting foods grown in the absence of chemical pesticides or selecting foods naturally low in toxins. To help ensure widespread safety, the Food and Drug Administration routinely tests both domestic and imported foods for pesticide residue and other potential toxins. A general program to minimize exposure to environmental and natural toxins includes knowing which foods pose greater risks, consuming a wide variety of

Table 13.2 Food-borne pathogens

Organism	Major sources	Symptoms	Onset	Estimated annual number of cases[a]
Bacteria				
Campylobacter jejuni	Raw poultry and meat, unpasteurized milk	Diarrhea, bloody stools, abdominal cramps, fever, headache. Lasts 7–10 days	2–5 days	2.0 million
Salmonella species	Raw meats, poultry, eggs, milk and dairy products, seafood, sauces and salad dressing	Nausea, vomiting, abdominal cramps, diarrhea, fever, headache. Lasts 1–2 days	6–48 hours	1.3 million
Clostridium perfringens	Meats, meat products, gravies, deep-dish casseroles	Intense abdominal cramps, diarrhea, nausea, fever. Lasts 6–24 hours	8–22 hours	249,000
Staphylococcus aureus (toxin)	Meat and meat products; poultry and egg products; salads such as egg, tuna, chicken, potato, and macaroni; cream-filled pastries; sandwich fillings; and milk and dairy products	Nausea, vomiting, retching, abdominal cramps, exhaustion. Lasts 1–2 days	30 minutes to 8 hours	185,000
Shigella species	Fecal contamination of food by unsanitary food handler	Abdominal cramps, diarrhea, fever, vomiting. Lasts 5–6 days	12 hours to 4 days	90,000
Escherichia coli O157:H7 (toxin)	Undercooked or raw ground beef, unpasteurized milk and fruit juices, raw vegetables	Abdominal pain, bloody diarrhea, colitus (intestinal bleeding), kidney failure. Lasts several days or weeks	5–48 hours	62,000
Listeria monocytogenes	Unpasteurized milk, soft cheeses, raw vegetables, sausages, raw and cooked poultry, raw meats, raw and smoked fish	Nausea, vomiting, diarrhea, fever, headache, stiff neck, chills. Pregnant women and fetuses are particularly susceptible. Leads to other complications such as meningitis. Can last weeks	Days to weeks	2,500 (high death rate)

	Source	Symptoms	Onset	Cases per year
Clostridium botulinum (toxin)	Home-canned foods, meat and seafood products, honey, commercially canned vegetables	Weakness, vertigo, double vision, difficulty swallowing, respiratory failure. Lasts several days	4–36 hours	<100 (high death rate)
Vibrio vulnificus	Raw seafood, especially oysters	Nausea, vomiting, diarrhea, fever, chills, abdominal cramps. Lasts 2–4 days	6–24 hours	<100 (high death rate)
Viruses				
Norwalk virus	Fecal contamination of food by unsanitary food handler; shellfish from contaminated water; salads and sandwiches	Nausea, vomiting, diarrhea, abdominal cramps, headache. Lasts 2–5 days	1–2 days	9.2 million
Hepatitis A virus	Fecal contamination of food by unsanitary food handler; shellfish from contaminated water	Fever, malaise, nausea, anorexia, and abdominal cramps, followed in several days by jaundice and possible liver damage. Lasts weeks to months	10–50 days	4,200
Protozoa				
Giardia lamblia	Fecal contamination of water and food	Abdominal cramps, diarrhea, nausea. Lasts 1–2 weeks, but chronic infections may last months to years	1–3 days	200,000
Taxoplasma gondii	Undercooked meat, unwashed fruits and vegetables	Flu-like symptoms, rash, diarrhea. In pregnant women, can cause spontaneous abortions and severe birth defects. Can last months	10–20 days	112,500
Cryptosporidium parvum	Fecal contamination of food by unsanitary food handler	Profuse watery diarrhea. Lasts days to weeks	1–12 days	30,000
Anisakis simplex	Raw fish	Severe abdominal pain. Can last months	1 hour to 2 weeks	<100
Trichinella spiralis	Undercooked pork and game meat	Muscle weakness, flu-like symptoms. Can last months	Weeks	<100

[a] From the Centers for Disease Control and Prevention (http://www.cdc.gov/ncidod/EID/vol5no5/mead.htm). Values represent yearly averages of data collected between 1983 and 1997.

foods, thoroughly rinsing fruits and vegetables, trimming fat from meat and poultry (including the skin), and discarding any fat that is rendered from meat, poultry, or fish during cooking.

Topic 13.3

Food Labeling

> **Key Points**
>
> Why do we need detailed food labels?
> What information is required on food labels?
> What additional information is allowed on food labels?

In response to consumer demand, the **Nutrition Labeling and Education Act of 1990** was created to give consumers detailed information about the nutrient content of food products. The food labels currently used in the United States are designed to help consumers make food-purchasing decisions and to plan their diets wisely. According to the regulations, virtually all food products that contain more than one ingredient must display the following information:

- The common name of the product
- The name and address of the manufacturer, packager, or distributor
- The amount of the product, expressed as weight, volume, or count
- The date by which the product should be sold
- The ingredients, listed in descending order of predominance by weight
- The nutrient content, presented in a specially designed "Nutrition Facts" panel

Additional voluntary information regarding the product's nutritive or health value may be included, but these claims must follow strict criteria. Small packages are allowed to contain some product information in abbreviated form or simply a phone number where the information can be found. Fresh fruits, vegetables, meat, fish, and poultry do not have to be individually labeled, although their nutrient content can be found on placards or pamphlets in many grocery stores. Most food served in restaurants, delicatessens, and bakeries is exempt from labeling.

An **ingredients list** is required for foods that contain more than one ingredient. The order in which they are listed must reflect their contribution to the total weight of the product. Anything that is intentionally put into the food must appear on the ingredients list, including natural and artificial food additives. Foods fortified with vitamins and minerals must indicate on the ingredients list the chemical form in which the vitamins and minerals were added. For example, vitamin C may appear on the label as either sodium ascorbate or ascorbic acid, depending on which chemical form was used in the manufacturing process.

The **Nutrition Facts** panel was designed to provide the energy and nutrient content found in a typical serving of the food (figure 13.1). The law requires that specific information be included regarding (i) the exact serving size and the number of servings per container, (ii) the number of Calories per serving and the number of Calories just from fat, and (iii) the amount per serving of the following nutrients:

- Total fat
- Saturated fat

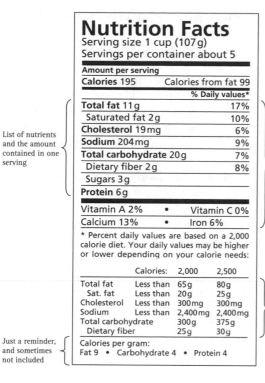

Figure 13.1   The Nutrition Facts Panel. The Nutrition Labeling and Education Act of 1990 requires that food products sold in the United States display nutrient information for consumer use.

- Cholesterol
- Sodium
- Total carbohydrate
- Dietary fiber
- Sugars
- Protein

In addition, the Nutrition Facts panel shows how the quantity of each nutrient compares to the nutrients' recommended daily amounts. The latter information is expressed as the % **daily value** and is intended to show how the food fits into an overall diet plan. Notice in figure 13.1 that only % daily values are required for vitamin A, vitamin C, calcium, and iron, whereas the % daily values are not required for sugars or protein.

The % daily values are perhaps the most confusing part of the Nutrition Facts panel. In order to make the percentage calculations, a daily **reference** amount must be established for each nutrient. The reference amount for vitamin A, vitamin C, calcium, and iron is based on the National Academy of Sciences' 1968 Recommended Dietary Allowances (RDAs). But no RDA exists for fat, cholesterol, sodium, carbohydrate, or fiber. Therefore, reference amounts for these nutrients are based on dietary guidelines for individuals consuming a 2,000-Calorie diet. For example, the current Dietary Guidelines for Americans recommends limiting fat intake to 30% of Calories. For a person consuming a 2,000-Calorie diet, this means that 600 Calories (30% of 2,000) would be provided by dietary fat. This roughly translates into 65 grams of fat, which is the reference amount shown in the bottom portion of figure 13.1. Each of the % daily values in the top portion of the Nutrition Facts panel are calculated from the reference amounts listed in the bottom portion. Also listed are reference amounts for a 2,500-Calorie diet for individuals who wish to calculate their own % daily values based on a higher energy diet.

The 1990 Nutrition Labeling and Education Act also allows food manufacturers to make nutritive or health claims about their product, as long as the claims abide by very strict criteria. For example, in order for a food to be called "fat free," it cannot contain more than 0.5 grams of fat per serving. Another example is the claim that a food is an "excellent source of" a particular nutrient. In this case, the food must provide 20% or more of the daily value for that nutrient. Certain health claims are allowed, such as "Excellent source of calcium . . . helps reduce the risk of osteoporosis." However, no health claim can be made if a food is high in total fat, saturated fat, cholesterol, or sodium.

Other products that require special label information are organic foods, irradiated foods, and dietary supplements. Foods are considered **organic** if they have been grown and processed without the use of synthetic pesticides, fertilizers, or additives. Organic crops cannot be grown on land that has been treated with synthetic chemicals within 3 years, and organic farmers must summit a plan and be certified by an agency overseen by the US Department of Agriculture. **Irradiation** is used to preserve and sterilize foods by killing insects, bacteria and other microorganisms. Irradiation is currently approved for use on poultry, meats, fresh fruit and vegetables, grains, and spices. Despite popular belief, irradiation does not make food radioactive, just as receiving a chest X-ray does not make your body radioactive. Irradiation has proven to be an effective way of controlling the growth of *Escherichia coli* and other pathogens in food. The labeling requirements of **dietary supplements** are discussed in Chapter 4.

Topic 13.4

Functional Foods

Key Points

What is a functional food?
What are the benefits and dangers associated with the consumption of functional foods?
To what extent is the manufacture and sale of functional foods regulated in the United States?

Decades ago, a food "product" was something people made at home with ingredients raised on the family farm or with "dry goods" purchased from the general store. Only in the past few years have foods been available to consumers as pre-made, pre-cooked, ready-to-eat products. These products have been developed by food manufacturers to meet consumer demand for convenience, taste, and value. More recently, increased consumer awareness of the link between diet and chronic diseases such as cancer and heart disease has created a demand for food and beverage products that also provide health benefits beyond the basic nutrient requirements of the body. The margarines Benecol and Take Control are examples of such products. These margarines are made with natural substances from plants that effectively lower blood cholesterol levels, yet Benecol and Take Control look and taste like regular margarine. Other examples include "trendy" soft drinks and "energy" bars that have herbs and other botanicals added to them. The terms **functional food** and **nutraceutical** are often used interchangeably to describe these products, although most experts prefer to use only the term "functional food," reserving "nutraceutical" for describing the specific substance used to make the functional food.

Another area of interest is the development of foods containing **probiotics** and **prebiotics**. About 200 different species of bacteria normally live in the human gastrointestinal tract, primarily in the large intestine. Considered "friendly" bacteria, they participate in intestinal metabolism and comprise about one-third the weight of fecal matter. Intestinal bacteria are capable of making several vitamins and immunoglobulins, although their most critical function is protection against infection and growth of pathogenic bacteria. The term probiotic is given to viable bacteria that exist in foods and have beneficial effects when ingested. Yogurt is an example of a probiotic food. Yogurt is made by fermenting milk with bacterial cultures, usually *Streptococcus thermophilus* or *Lactobacillus bulgaricus*. Food manufacturers have developed several dairy products with additional probiotics such as *Bifidobacterium lactis*, *Lactobacillus acidophilus*, and other *Lactobacillus* bacteria. Another way of "delivering" probiotics to the large intestine is by ingesting supplements (such as capsules) containing viable bacteria.

In contrast to probiotics, a prebiotic is a nutrient that is utilized by the beneficial bacteria in the gastrointestinal tract. The most widely recognized prebiotics are indigestible carbohydrates that are unavailable for absorption and pass into the large intestine. Fructooligosaccharide (FOS) and inulin (not to be confused with insulin) are among the most popular prebiotics currently being marketed. FOS is a sucrose molecule linked to one, two, or three fructose molecules. It can be purchased by food manufacturers in syrup or crystalline form for incorporation into food products. Inulin is a long chain of fructose units and is found mostly in chicory root and Jerusalem artichokes. Wheatgerm and honey can also influence the growth of intestinal bacterial and are currently being investigated for their prebiotic potential.

Using food as therapy is not new. Ancient cultures often used foods to treat illness or to alter mood. Only in the past few years have scientists begun to identify the specific chemicals in food that provide the purported health benefits. Food manufacturers have capitalized on this information by incorporating the isolated chemicals into their product recipes, thus creating the functional food industry. A long list of "beneficial" substances has been identified, the majority of which are **phytochemicals** found naturally in plants (table 13.3). While the concept of functional foods has merit, the actual health benefits they provide are sometimes difficult to determine because of the long-term nature of chronic diseases. Nevertheless, many people feel that even in the absence of scientific evidence, functional foods provide consumers with greater food choices in planning a healthful diet. However, there are opponents who claim that concentrating a single chemical and putting it into a food can increase health risks. They argue that consuming the diverse array of phytochemicals in the amounts normally found in food is relatively safe, but that large doses of one substance could produce toxic side effects. They also argue that adding phytochemicals to foods such as candy bars and snack foods could mislead consumers into believing that any food made into a functional food will promote health.

Although these concerns are debatable, they do raise the issue of whether functional foods—because of the addition of specific chemical substances—should be considered a type of drug. According to the Food, Drug, and Cosmetic Act of 1938, **drugs** are substances that "diagnose, treat, prevent, cure, or mitigate disease." This definition is precisely how many people view functional foods, even though a universally accepted definition has not yet been established. It could be argued that the only difference between drugs and functional foods is that drugs contain chemical substances in isolated form, whereas functional foods contain the chemicals within a food "carrier." From this point of view, there does not appear to be a clear distinction between drugs and functional foods. This issue becomes even less definitive when one considers that many of our modern drugs are based on substances found in nature, and that substances added to functional foods are also natural substances normally found in the food supply. In some cases, a product could be both a functional food and a drug if it is designed and represented for both uses.

Table 13.3 Some phytochemicals and their food sources

Class or name	Food sources
Allium compounds	Onions, garlic, chives, leeks
Capsaicin	Hot peppers
Carotenoids (includes beta-carotene and lycopene)	Yellow/orange fruits and vegetables, dark green leafy vegetables
Coumarins	Vegetables and citrus fruits
Flavonoids (includes isoflavones and catechin)	Most fruits and vegetables, whole wheat, wine, green tea, black tea
Indoles	Cruciferous vegetables
Isothiocyanates	Cruciferous vegetables
Lignans	Whole grains
Monoterpenes (includes limonene)	Citrus fruits peels and oils
Phenols	Most fruits and vegetables, green tea, coffee beans
Phytic acid	Whole grains
Phytosterols	Most legumes (particularly soybeans)
Saponins	Most vegetables
Tannins	Legumes, wine, tea

So where do we draw the line between a "functional food" and a "drug?" The answer lies mainly in their legal definitions and the laws that govern their manufacture and sale. In the United States, the use of the term "drug" has traditionally meant **substances other than food**. Therefore, the manufacture and sale of drugs is subject to regulations that do not necessarily apply to food. Makers of functional foods can avoid many of the regulations imposed on drug manufacturers by selecting substances that have little or no restrictions, such as herbs and other botanicals. The loose regulations that currently govern the use of "natural substances" in functional foods as well as dietary supplements have fueled much debate on their potential toxicity. Many experts believe that a more rigorous review process should be imposed on new products in a manner similar to the pharmaceutical industry. The result of the loose regulations is that many new functional foods that have undergone virtually no testing or safety evaluation are popping up on grocery store shelves. Furthermore, food manufacturers are also allowed to make health claims as long as the following appears on the food label: *"This statement has not been evaluated by the Food and Drug Administration. This product is not intended to diagnose, treat, cure or prevent any disease."* The lack of specific regulations has led many consumer groups to call for tighter laws regarding the manufacture and sale of functional foods.

The "gray area" surrounding the definition and application of functional foods has placed a greater responsibility on consumers to understand the benefits and potential dangers associated with functional foods. Any chemical substance in food can be toxic if ingested in excessive amounts, yet when consumed in reasonable amounts, the same chemical can influence the body's metabolism in beneficial ways. The next few years will undoubtedly bring increasing regulations on how much of a specific substance will be allowed in functional foods and what specific health claims can be made. In the meantime, consumers should not view functional foods as a substitute for medical treatment or as a quick fix for an existing illness. Choosing whether to consume functional foods should be based on credible information and on how well functional foods fit into an individual's long-term dietary plan.

Application

Organic foods have become very popular in recent years because of the belief that they are healthy and safer than the "processed" foods found in most supermarkets. However, like many issues in nutrition, a common understanding of organic foods is often lacking among consumers. The US Department of Agriculture has recently developed tighter standards for the production and marketing of organic foods. In addition to the current definition of having no synthetic pesticides, fertilizers, or additives during production, the new regulations prohibit the use of genetic engineering, irradiation, and sewage sludge as a fertilizer. But do these strict requirements produce a healthier, safer food? In terms of nutrient content, the answer is "no." Organic fruits, vegetables, grains, nuts, and meats have the same nutrient composition as their nonorganic counterparts. In terms of pathogen exposure and food-borne illness, the answer is also "no." Organic and nonorganic foods are the same when it comes to their ability to support the growth of dangerous microorganisms. Organic foods are usually processed under the same conditions as nonorganic foods using the same equipment and workers, so the opportunity to contaminate or cross-contaminate is identical. One could argue that because organic foods cannot undergo irradiation to kill microorganisms, they could prove to be a greater risk than nonorganic foods in some cases. Finally, in terms of chemical residues, the answer is "it depends." It depends on each person's level of tolerance and personal preference. Scientifically, the amount of pesticide residue on nonorganic foods is generally so low that no toxic or carcinogenic effects have been detected in laboratory tests (which is why their use is approved in the United States). Some people, however, prefer to live by a zero tolerance standard and will select organic foods whenever possible.

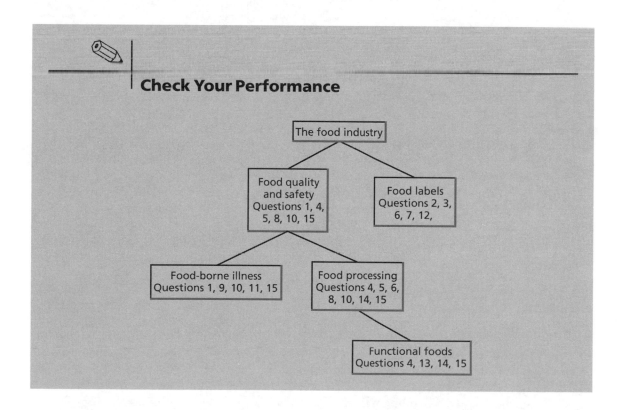

Check Your Performance

Chapter Test

True/False
1. Washing your hands before and during food preparation can be an effective way to decrease the risk of food-borne illness
2. The % Daily Value used on the Nutritional Facts panel is based on the typical American diet of 4,000 Calories per day
3. Most food served in restaurants, delicatessens, and bakeries is exempt from labeling
4. Phytochemicals are substances naturally found in plants that, when ingested, can cause severe illness and death
5. Irradiation is an effective way to increase the shelf life of certain foods

Multiple Choice
6. The production, processing, and distribution of "organic" foods is regulated by
    a. The National Institutes of Health
    b. The US Department of Agriculture
    c. The Food and Drug Administration
    d. The Centers for Disease Control and Prevention
7. Which of the following food products is *not* required to have a complete Nutrition Facts panel?
    a. Can of vegetable soup
    b. One pound tub of margarine
    c. Bite-sized candy bar
    d. Large loaf of whole wheat bread
8. Which of the following food processing methods is *not* based on temperature treatment?
    a. Fermentation
    b. Pasteurization
    c. Canning
    d. Sterilization
9. The incidence of food-borne illness in the United States is most often caused by
    a. Pesticide residue
    b. Viruses
    c. Pathogenic bacteria
    d. Industrial contaminants
10. Which of the following food additives is most likely to inhibit the growth of microorganisms?
    a. Lecithin
    b. Folic acid
    c. Monosodium glutamate
    d. Salt

Short Answer
11. What is the difference between food-borne infection and food-borne intoxication?
12. Why does the US government require food labels?
13. What is a functional food?
14. Describe at least three examples of whole foods fortified with nutrients not normally found in significant amounts

Essay
15. Describe some important ways in which food processing techniques improve the safety, wholesomeness, and availability of food

Further Reading

American Dietetic Association (1999) Position of the American Dietetic Association: functional foods. *Journal of the American Dietetic Association*, **99**, 1278–85.

Bremner, H.A. (2000) Toward practical definitions of quality for food science. *Critical Reviews in Food Science and Nutrition*, **40**, 83–90.

Hasler, C.M. (2000) The changing face of functional foods. *Journal of the American College of Nutrition*, **19**(Suppl. 5), 499S–506S.

Levy, L., Patterson, R.E., Kristal, A.R. & Li, S.S. (2000) How well do consumers understand percentage daily value on food labels? *American Journal of Health Promotion*, **14**, 157–60.

Lucas, C.D., Hallagan, J.B. & Taylor, S.L. (2001) The role of natural color additives in food allergy. *Advances in Food and Nutrition Research*, **43**, 195–216.

Prosky, L. (2000) When is dietary fiber considered a functional food? *Biofactors*, **12**, 289–97.

Sloan, A.E. (1996) America's appetite: the top 10 trends to watch and work on. *Food Technology*, **50**(7), 55–71.

Tritsch, G.L. (2000) Food irradiation. *Nutrition*, **16**, 698–701.

Williams, P.R. & Hammitt, J.K. (2001) Perceived risks of conventional and organic produce: pesticides, pathogens, and natural toxins. *Risk Analysis*, **21**, 319–30.

Wood, O.B. & Bruhn, C.M. (2000) Position of the American Dietetic Association: food irradiation. *Journal of the American Dietetic Association*, **100**, 246–53.

Worthington, V. (1998) Effects of agricultural methods on nutritional quality: a comparison of organic with conventional crops. *Alternative Therapies in Health and Medicine*, **4**, 58–69.

Chapter 14

A Healthy Future

Factors known to influence a person's long-term health include genetics, diet, and physical activity. While we humans have little control over our genes, we do have control over what we eat and how physically active we are. Previous chapters have focused primarily on how diet is related to overall health and well being, but staying physically active can be just as important to long-term health. This chapter highlights some metabolic aspects of exercise and briefly discusses the benefits of staying physically active. In addition, this chapter includes a discussion on the concept of "optimal health." Despite the widespread use of the term "optimal" among health professionals, there does not seem to be widespread consensus on its intended meaning. Resource information is also provided for readers wishing to further explore nutrition-related topics that can help in planning for a healthy future.

Essential Background

❖ Understanding the purpose of dietary standards and dietary guidelines (Chapter 4)
❖ Energy capture and utilization by the body (Chapter 5)
❖ Energy balance and body composition (Chapter 8)
❖ The relationships between nutrition and chronic diseases (Chapter 9)

Topic 14.1

Physical Activity

> **Key Points**
>
> How does physical activity contribute to health?
> What energy sources provide fuel for muscle movement?
> How does the type of exercise affect what fuels will be used? And how is oxygen involved?
> What are the dietary recommendations for physically active people?

Health care professionals use the term **fitness** to describe how well an individual can perform physical activity. **Exercise** can be thought of as planned or structured physical activity intended to improve physical fitness. Regular exercise provides many health benefits, including decreased risk of heart disease, osteoporosis, and some types of cancer. Exercise also "burns" energy and helps the body stay in energy balance, thus reducing the risk of obesity. In this way, exercise reduces the risk of obesity-related conditions such as diabetes mellitus, coronary heart disease, and hypertension (see Chapter 9). People who exercise also claim to have reduced stress and anxiety, as well as improved sleeping and mental function. Furthermore, regular exercise benefits the cardiovascular and respiratory systems by increasing the efficiency of oxygen transport in the blood. This means that the heart muscle becomes stronger and pumps more blood with each beat, which, in turn, slows the resting pulse rate and increases breathing efficiency.

The benefits of exercise are indisputable, yet many people find it difficult to fit exercise into their daily routine. It is important to recognize that a person does not need to be an athlete to reap the benefits of exercise. Many studies have shown that even a little bit of exercise is better than no exercise. Simply taking the stairs instead of the elevator or parking your car further away from the store entrance can mean increased physical activity for some people. One of the main focuses of the Dietary Guidelines for Americans 2000 is to "Aim for Fitness," as described in Chapter 4. The Guidelines advise people to:

- Engage in at least 30 minutes (adults) or 60 minutes (children) of moderate physical activity most, preferably all, days of the week
- Become physically active if you are inactive
- Maintain or increase physical activity if you are already active
- Stay active throughout your life
- Help children get at least 60 minutes of physical activity daily
- Choose physical activities that fit in with your daily routine, or choose recreational or structured exercise programs, or both
- Consult your health care provider before starting a new vigorous physical activity plan if you have a chronic health problem, or if you are over 40 (men) or 50 (women)

These recommendations may seem intimidating to someone who is just getting started in a regular exercise routine. Keep in mind that these are general guidelines aimed at the whole population. Each person will need to consider his or her individual lifestyle and personal goals when planning a long-term exercise program. Virtually everyone can gain some sort of health benefit by increasing physical activity, as long as the activity is reasonable and achievable.

The nutrients that are used for energy to fuel muscle activity are primarily glucose (from the diet or glycogen stores) and fatty acids (from the diet or triglyceride stores). Amino acids from protein may also be used for energy, but the amount used is very small compared to glucose and fatty acids. The body uses varying proportions of both glucose and fatty acids during physical activity depending on the **intensity** and **duration** of the activity. When at rest, the body uses mostly fatty acids for energy. As the intensity of muscle activity increases, glucose from muscle glycogen becomes the predominate energy source because glucose is more immediately available to the muscle than fatty acids. Conserving muscle glycogen when at rest is the body's way of having enough reserve energy for quick action in times of emergency. Consequently, short-duration, high-intensity activities such as sprinting, jumping, or lifting weights use nearly 100% glucose for energy. Moderate activities such as walking or gardening use a mixture of fatty acids and glucose. As the intensity of physical activity increases, the ability to maintain that activity decreases because of the limited availability of glucose—the body's glucose reserves are much less than the body's fat reserves. However just because low-intensity activities use fatty acids for energy, don't be misled into thinking that sitting in front of the television will promote body fat loss. One must increase *total* energy expenditure relative to energy intake in order to lose excess body fat (see Chapter 8). A person who exercises by walking must walk for 1 hour to burn the same amount of energy as someone who runs for 20 minutes.

Inside the muscle cell, all fuels—whether glucose, fatty acids, or amino acids—must transfer their energy to adenosine triphosphate (ATP) in order for the cell to use the energy. Recall from Chapter

3 that ATP is the "energy broker" for most body functions. The amount of ATP that is present in muscle cells at any point in time is actually quite small, so ATP must be continually regenerated. If ATP was not replenished, there would only be enough for about 10 seconds of muscle movement. Even though glucose from glycogen can quickly regenerate ATP, high-intensity activities may require more ATP than glucose can provide. Fortunately, muscle cells have a back-up system that involves another "high energy" molecule called **phosphocreatine**. There is about five times more phosphocreatine in muscle than ATP, and although phosphocreatine cannot be used directly for energy, it can replenish ATP more quickly than glucose. Phosphocreatine, like ATP, ultimately receives its energy from glucose, fatty acids, or amino acids. Although phosphocreatine is made from creatine in the body, some athletes believe that taking **creatine supplements** can increase the amount of phosphocreatine in muscle and therefore enhance athletic performance. While studies have shown that creatine supplements can indeed increase phosphocreatine in muscle, their effect on athletic performance is debatable.

The type of fuel used during physical activity also depends on the efficiency with which oxygen is delivered to muscle cells. Oxygen must be present to metabolize fatty acids and amino acids—without oxygen, these fuel sources cannot be used to make ATP. However, glucose can regenerate a small amount of ATP in the absence of oxygen, but a much larger amount of ATP will be made from glucose if oxygen is present. The complete breakdown of glucose, fatty acids, or amino acids to yield ATP when oxygen is present is called **aerobic metabolism**. Someone who is physically fit or "in shape" has developed an increased capacity to deliver oxygen to muscle cells and will therefore make ATP more efficiently through aerobic metabolism. But in times when muscle activity is required and oxygen levels are insufficient, the body will make limited amounts of ATP from glucose through **anaerobic metabolism**. When oxygen is unavailable, glucose breakdown is incomplete and results in the formation of **lactic acid**. Accumulation of lactic acid is thought to cause sore muscles in someone who is "out of shape." Stopping occasionally during exercise to replenish the oxygen supply can minimize lactic acid accumulation. Lactic acid can eventually be used for fuel via aerobic metabolism or used by the liver to make glucose via gluconeogenesis.

Exercise does increase the body's total energy expenditure. This is good news for someone wishing to lose excess body fat, but a person who is maintaining body weight will need to increase energy intake to stay in energy balance. Fortunately, exercise generally requires no special diet. Physically active people can meet their nutrient needs by following the dietary recommendations for the general population as outlined by the Food Guide Pyramid (see Chapter 4). The only adjustment is that exercisers may need to focus on the upper range of the serving size recommendations to meet their energy needs. Exercise also increases the need for vitamins and minerals that function in energy metabolism. Consuming a well-balanced diet based on the Food Guide Pyramid will meet these increased needs for most people. A vitamin and mineral supplement may be necessary for physically active people who consume a low-energy diet or competitive athletes such as gymnastics or wrestlers who often restrict their nutrient intake.

Topic 14.2

The Concept of "Optimal Health"

Key Points

What is health?
Can health be optimized?
How do we achieve optimal health?

Most people want to be healthy. We are willing to change our diets, exercise more, and even try unconventional therapies to achieve good health. Yet, as we strive to be more healthy, we seldom stop to think about what we mean by the term "health." Defining health may not be as simple as it first appears, perhaps because health is more than just a physical condition. A complete understanding of health encompasses all aspects of a person's well being, including his or her mental, social, and even spiritual condition. When approached from this holistic point of view, one can imagine all of the many factors that might contribute to a person's overall health.

The culture in which we live not only has a direct influence on a person's health, it also influences our perception of health. People living in Western societies such as the United States tend to view health from a **scientific perspective**. That is, we have come to depend on science to explain many things about nature, including issues related to health. Consider that our modern health care system involves training physicians (including psychiatrists) to identify conditions of ill health and then to formulate an appropriate treatment based on scientific research. In other words, the primary focus of science-based health care is to treat disease. Consequently, the definition of health in Western societies tends to be based on the absence or presence of disease; one might say they are in "good health" if they are free of disease.

Some people find this science-based definition of good health to be too limited. Indeed, subtle changes in a person's health can occur even in the absence of disease. Expanding our definition, therefore, requires us to look at health from non-scientific viewpoints. There are, in fact, cultures around the world that employ non-scientific systems of medicine that have fundamentally different perspectives of health than we are accustomed to in Western societies. For example, **ayurveda** is a way of life in India and has been practiced for more than 4,000 years. Ayurveda teaches that life and health depend on the proper balance of the senses, mind, body, and soul. Another example is **traditional Chinese medicine (TCM)**, which is a system of health care that is more than 2,000 years old. TCM is based on principles of balance and countermeasures that strive to keep the body's opposing energies (called Yin and Yang) in balance and flowing properly through the body's energy pathways (called meridians). Unlike the "disease-identification-and-treatment" approach of modern medicine, these ancient systems of health care focus on achieving and maintaining **wellness**. Ayurveda and TCM are able to detect subtle states of imbalance within an individual well before these imbalances manifest themselves as a clinical disease.

When viewed from the ancients' perspective, it would seem no single definition of good health is satisfactory for every individual under every circumstance. Although some people may simply view good health as a physical condition in which disease is absent, most people believe **good health** is a state of physical *and* mental well being that can fluctuate and have varying degrees of "good." Recognizing that a person's state of well being can fluctuate within the range of good health is central to understanding the concept of **optimal health**.

The fact that other cultures base their understanding of health on holistic observations raises the question of whether biomedical science—with all its marvelous technology—can provide information about optimal health. Recall from Chapter 12 that the scientific method is only applicable to situations where disease exists and where indicators of health (such as blood pressure) can be measured in tangible ways. The scientific method becomes less useful when disease is not present or when we consider health and wellness in more subjective, intangible terms that have no objective measurable indicators of health. For example, a TCM practitioner will feel the pulse of a patient to diagnose states of imbalance or well being. In contrast to science-based medicine, where pulse is understood in terms of rate or strength, Chinese pulse theory distinguishes some 28 pulse types—such as hollow, scattered, wiry, soggy, confined, etc.—that offer a subtle expression of underlying health or disharmony. In this sense, both ayurveda and TCM seem better suited than science to assess the **quality** of a person's health *in the absence of disease*. These ancient systems of health care have long recognized optimal health as something unique and achievable in every person; however, scientists have not yet been able to find an objective, physical measurement that reflects "optimal" health for every person.

Recognizing the **limitations** of biomedical science in defining optimal health should in no way detract from the vital role science has played in helping us understand how the body functions. Scientific research has allowed us to understand diet and disease relationships in ways that no other approach can provide. Discovery of the vitamins in the early part of the twentieth century, for example, established the concept of "essential nutrient" and thus helped eliminate many deficiency diseases that were once common throughout the world. We have also learned from science that certain dietary substances can influence chronic diseases. Some have argued that the scientific discoveries of the past century have improved the quality of human life more than any other factor. But the contributions from science in defining an individual's level of wellness will always be confined to those aspects of health that can only be addressed by the scientific method.

So, how should we view "optimal health"? Clearly, no universal definition would be appropriate for all people. The ancient systems of health care have taught us that optimal health is a state of wellness unique to every individual and that no single standard of measurement would be appropriate for every person. It's also apparent that the one-size-fits-all dietary recommendations used in Western societies, while useful in promoting health on a population basis, does not adequately address optimal health for all individuals. Striving for optimal health, therefore, requires us to take responsibility for our own health and to learn the subtle ways in which our health can change even in the absence of disease. Science-based dietary recommendations can point us toward adequate diets that prevent nutrient deficiencies and lower the risk of chronic diseases, but fine-tuning good health requires a broader understanding of nutrition that ventures beyond the confines of science.

Topic 14.3

Information Resources

> **Key Points**
>
> Who are the nutrition experts?
> Where can you find reliable nutrition information?
> What career opportunities are there in the nutrition field?

Finding reliable nutrition information can be a challenge, particularly in free market societies where fraud and quackery are prevalent. Confounding the problem is the growing desire of consumers to learn more about the non-scientific ("alternative") aspects of nutrition and health. This leaves the door open for "experts" to promote just about any half-baked idea that sounds somewhat convincing. Moreover, the title of "nutrition expert" can be claimed by anyone, with or without experience in nutrition and health. In the United States, scientific nutrition information is generally reliable if it comes from registered dietitians, nutrition professors, pharmacists, public health professionals, and physicians.

Registered dietitians (RDs) are food and nutrition professionals who have fulfilled the requirements established by the American Dietetic Association (ADA). To earn the RD credential, a person must complete a minimum of a bachelor's degree with specific courses in food and nutrition sciences, foodservice systems management, business, economics, educational psychology, chemistry, biochemistry, microbiology, anatomy, and physiology. In addition, a person must complete a 6–12-month supervised practice program (internship) at a health care facility, community agency, or a foodservice corporation. Finally, they must pass the national examination administered by the ADA. Each year they must also complete continuing professional educational requirements to maintain registration.

Nutrition professors generally hold doctoral degrees in nutrition or a closely related field such as biochemistry or food science. Part of their education includes extensive training in research, and many seek out post-doctoral research positions before becoming professors. **Pharmacists** also receive some training in the nutrition area and should be able to answer questions regarding drug–nutrient interactions. A number of **public health professionals** can be found in the government section of the telephone directory. You may need to search local, state, and federal agencies to find the best qualified person to provide the information you seek. While many people look to their **physicians** for dietary advice, only about one-fourth of all medical schools in the United States required even one course in nutrition. Physicians generally need to educate themselves about nutrition issues once they have established a medical practice. There are, however, some physicians who specialize in nutrition-related disorders.

Notice that the title "nutritionist" is not used by most bone fide professionals. This is because the terms "nutritionist," "nutritionalist," "nutripathist," and the like are somewhat vague and are often used by unqualified individuals who flaunt bogus credentials. There are a number of fraudulent correspondence schools that "award" bogus nutrition certificates—for a fee, of course. The documents provided by these diploma mills often have impressive sounding affiliations: "The International Academy of Nutrition Consultants" or "The American Association of Nutrition Therapists." These particular institutions, however, do not exist. If you have questions regarding the legitimacy of mail order "institutions," you should contact the American Dietetic Association for verification.

Individuals with proper training in nutrition or dietetics have a number of career options available to them. Hospitals, corporations, schools, and other institutions employ qualified individuals in positions of foodservice management, food production, and nutrition counseling. Some institutions have developed wellness programs that are directed by experienced nutrition professionals. Public health and volunteer agencies employ qualified individuals to develop nutrition education programs and literature. In addition, many undergraduate students interested in medical, dental, and other health professional careers are choosing nutrition majors with increasing frequency.

For further information regarding nutrition and health and career opportunities, the internet offers a direct link to health organizations, universities, and government agencies. As mentioned in Chapter 12, caution should be exercised when accessing commercial websites that promote the sale of products or diet plans. Table 14.1 provides contact information for several reliable websites.

Application

Despite the benefits associated with exercise, most Americans do not have a regular exercise routine. Studies have shown that about half of the individuals who start a personal exercise program quit within 6 months. Initial interest in exercise is usually related to a desire to be healthy, although that initial enthusiasm can fade as the reality of our daily lives thwarts our best intentions. It appears that *how* a person gets started can influence how well an exercise routine is maintained over the long term. Studies have shown that the exercise habits of adults are often established in childhood. School exercise programs, in addition to their impact on the health and fitness of children, can provide the enjoyment and knowledge about exercise that clearly affects

Table 14.1 Nutrition information resources

Institution/organization	Contact information
US Department of Agriculture, Food and Nutrition Information Center	www.nal.usda.gov/fnic
US Department of Health and Human Services	www.os.dhhs.gov
National Center for Complementary and Alternative Medicine	www.nccam.nih.gov
Food and Drug Administration	www.fda.gov
FDA Center for Food Safety and Applied Nutrition	www.cfsan.fda.gov
Centers for Disease Control and Prevention	www.cdc.gov
National Institutes of Health	www.nih.gov/health
Consumer Information Center	www.pueblo.gsa.gov
American Dietetic Association	www.eatright.org
American Medical Association	www.ama-assn.org
International Food Information Council	www.ific.org
International Life Sciences Institute	www.ilsi.org
American Cancer Society	www.cancer.org
American Diabetes Association	www.diabetes.org
American Heart Association	www.americanheart.org
National Osteoporosis Foundation	www.nof.org
Mayo Clinic Health Information	www.mayohealth.org
Tufts University Nutrition Navigator	www.navigator.tufts.edu
National Eating Disorders Association	www.nationaleatingdisorders.org
National Association of Anorexia Nervosa and Associated Disorders	www.anad.org
World Health Organization (WHO)	www.who.org
Food and Agriculture Organization of the United Nations (FAO)	www.fao.org

future patterns of adherence. For adults who are not accustomed to exercise, the goal of 30 minutes per day may require some behavior change. Recognizing the reasons for not exercising is the first step. "Not enough time" is a common excuse, although finding 30 minutes in a 24-hour day is really not that much. A primary reason way most people don't exercise is due to a feeling of discomfort or lack of enjoyment. Finding an exercise program that is fun, such as exercising with a friend or following a video program, can improve the long-term success rate. Above all, create an exercise program that is right for you—a little exercise is better than none.

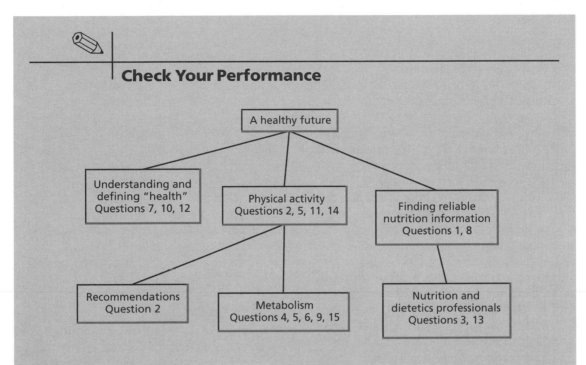

Check Your Performance

Chapter Test

True/False

1. The internet should be avoided when searching for reliable nutrition information because most credible organizations do not have websites

2. The Dietary Guidelines for Americans recommend that adults exercise 30 minutes per day and children exercise 60 minutes per day

3. A "nutritionist" is a person who holds a bachelor's degree and who passed the Nutritionists Academy national examination

4. Although their use is widespread, creatine supplements have not been proven to increase athletic performance

5. Anaerobic metabolism is less efficient than aerobic metabolism because it does not produce any ATP

Multiple Choice

6. What do glucose, fatty acids, and amino acids have in common?
   a. They are always found together in the same foods
   b. They are all used for energy to fuel muscle activity
   c. Each can be used to make ATP via anaerobic metabolism
   d. All of the above

7. What is Ayurveda?
   a. A type of aerobic exercise
   b. An herbal supplement sold only on the internet
   c. A way of life that strives for balance of the senses, mind, body, and soul
   d. None of the above

8. When searching for credible nutrition information, who is probably the least reliable resource?

    a. Pharmacist
    b. Public health official
    c. Registered dietitian
    d. Sales clerk at Universal Nutrition Center

9. What is phosphocreatine?
    a. A high-energy molecule similar to ATP
    b. A dietary supplement recommended for pregnant women
    c. An essential nutrient required in the human diet
    d. All of the above

10. Traditional Chinese Medicine
    a. Focuses on maintaining wellness and preventing illness
    b. Has been practiced for more than 2,000 years
    c. Strives to keep the body's opposing energies in balance
    d. All of the above

Short Answer

11. Define "fitness"
12. What is the relationship between "good health" and "optimal health"?
13. What is a registered dietitian?
14. How does exercise improve health?
15. What is aerobic metabolism?

Further Reading

Cheuvront, S.N. (1999) The zone diet and athletic performance. *Sports Medicine*, **27**, 213–28.

Chopra, A. & Doiphode, V.V. (2002) Ayurvedic medicine: core concept, therapeutic principles, and current relevance. *Medical Clinics of North America*, **86**, 75–89.

Clark, P.A. (2000) The ethics of alternative medicine therapies. *Journal of Public Health Policy*, **21**, 447–70.

Dietitians of Canada (2000) Position of Dietitians of Canada, the American Dietetic Association, and the American College of Sports Medicine: nutrition and athletic performance. *Canadian Journal of Dietetic Practice and Research*, **61**, 176–92.

Dodd, J.L. (1997) Incorporating genetics into dietary guidance. *Food Technology*, **51**(3), 80–2.

Gillman, M.W., Pinto, B.M., Tennstedt, S., Glanz, K., Marcus, B. & Friedman, R.H. (2001) Relationships of physical activity with dietary behaviors among adults. *Preventive Medicine*, **32**, 295–301.

Heimburger, D.C., Stallings, V.A. & Routzahn, L. (1998) Survey of clinical nutrition training programs for physicians. *American Journal of Clinical Nutrition*, **68**, 1174–9.

Jakicic, J.M., Clark, K., Coleman, E., *et al.* (2001) American College of Sports Medicine position stand. Appropriate intervention strategies for weight loss and prevention of weight regain for adults. *Medicine and Science in Sports and Exercise*, **33**, 2145–56.

Meisler, J.G. (2001) Toward optimal health: the experts discuss the American diet. *Journal of Women's Health & Gender-Based Medicine*, **10**, 519–23.

Nestler, G. (2002) Traditional Chinese medicine. *Medical Clinics of North America*, **86**, 63–73.

Sunday, J., Eyles, J. & Upshur, R. (2001) Applying Aristotle's doctrine of causation to Aboriginal and bio-medical understanding of diabetes. *Culture, Medicine and Psychiatry*, **25**, 63–85.

Twisk, J.W. (2001) Physical activity guidelines for children and adolescents: a critical review. *Sports Medicine*, **31**, 617–27.

Williams, M.H. (1999) *Nutrition For Health, Fitness & Sport*, 5th ed. WCB/McGraw-Hill, Boston.

Appendix A

Dietary Reference Intakes (DRIs)

Life stage group	Vitamin A (μg/d)[a]	Vitamin C (mg/d)	Vitamin D (μg/d)[b]	Vitamin E (mg/d)[c]	Vitamin K (μg/d)	Thiamin (mg/d)	Riboflavin (mg/d)	Niacin (mg/d)[d]	Vitamin B6 (mg/d)
Infants									
0–6 mo	400	40	5	4	2.0	0.2	0.3	2	0.1
7–12 mo	500	50	5	5	2.5	0.3	0.4	4	0.3
Children									
1–3 yr	300	15	5	6	30	0.5	0.5	6	0.5
4–8 yr	400	25	5	7	55	0.6	0.6	8	0.6
Males									
9–13 yr	600	45	5	11	60	0.9	0.9	12	1.0
14–18 yr	900	75	5	15	75	1.2	1.3	16	1.3
19–30 yr	900	90	5	15	120	1.2	1.3	16	1.3
31–50 yr	900	90	5	15	120	1.2	1.3	16	1.3
51–70 yr	900	90	10	15	120	1.2	1.3	16	1.7
>70 yr	900	90	15	15	120	1.2	1.3	16	1.7
Females									
9–13 yr	600	45	5	11	60	0.9	0.9	12	1.0
14–18 yr	700	65	5	15	75	1.0	1.0	14	1.2
19–30 yr	700	75	5	15	90	1.1	1.1	14	1.3
31–50 yr	700	75	5	15	90	1.1	1.1	14	1.3
51–70 yr	700	75	10	15	90	1.1	1.1	14	1.5
>70 yr	700	75	15	15	90	1.1	1.1	14	1.5
Pregnancy									
≤18 yr	750	80	5	15	75	1.4	1.4	18	1.9
19–30 yr	770	85	5	15	90	1.4	1.4	18	1.9
31–50 yr	770	85	5	15	90	1.4	1.4	18	1.9
Lactation									
≤18 yr	1,200	115	5	19	75	1.4	1.6	17	2.0
19–30 yr	1,300	120	5	19	90	1.4	1.6	17	2.0
31–50 yr	1,300	120	5	19	90	1.4	1.6	17	2.0

[a] As retinol activity equivalents (RAE).
[b] As calciferol.
[c] As α-tocopherol.
[d] As niacin equivalents (NE).

cont. p. 170

Life stage group	Folate (μg/d)[e]	Vitamin B_{12} (μg/d)	Pantothenic Acid (mg/d)	Biotin (μg/d)	Choline (mg/d)[f]	Calcium (mg/d)	Chromium (μg/d)	Copper (μg/d)	Fluoride (mg/d)
Infants									
0–6 mo	65	0.4	1.7	5	125	210	0.2	200	0.01
7–12 mo	80	0.5	1.8	6	150	270	5.5	220	0.5
Children									
1–3 yr	150	0.9	2	8	200	500	11	340	0.7
4–8 yr	200	1.2	3	12	250	800	15	440	1
Males									
9–13 yr	300	1.8	4	20	375	1,300	25	700	2
14–18 yr	400	2.4	5	25	550	1,300	35	890	3
19–30 yr	400	2.4	5	30	550	1,000	35	900	4
31–50 yr	400	2.4	5	30	550	1,000	35	900	4
51–70 yr	400	2.4[g]	5	30	550	1,200	30	900	4
>70 yr	400	2.4[g]	5	30	550	1,200	30	900	4
Females									
9–13 yr	300	1.8	4	20	375	1,300	21	700	2
14–18 yr	400[h]	2.4	5	25	400	1,300	24	890	3
19–30 yr	400[h]	2.4	5	30	425	1,000	25	900	3
31–50 yr	400[h]	2.4	5	30	425	1,000	25	900	3
51–70 yr	400	2.4[g]	5	30	425	1,200	20	900	3
>70 yr	400	2.4[g]	5	30	425	1,200	20	900	3
Pregnancy									
≤18 yr	600	2.6	6	30	450	1,300	29	1,000	3
19–30 yr	600	2.6	6	30	450	1,000	30	1,000	3
31–50 yr	600	2.6	6	30	450	1,000	30	1,000	3
Lactation									
≤18 yr	500	2.8	7	35	550	1,300	44	1,300	3
19–30 yr	500	2.8	7	35	550	1,000	45	1,300	3
31–50 yr	500	2.8	7	35	550	1,000	45	1,300	3

[e] As dietary folate equivalents (DFE).

[f] Although Adequate Intakes (AI) have been set for choline, there are few data to assess whether a dietary supply of choline is needed at all stages of the life cycle, and it may be that the choline requirement can be met by endogenous synthesis at some of these stages.

[g] Because 10–30 percent of older people may malabsorb food-bound vitamin B_{12}, it is advisable for those older than 50 years to meet their RDA mainly by consuming foods fortified with vitamin B_{12} or a supplement containing vitamin B_{12}.

[h] In view of the evidence linking folate intake with neural tube defects in the fetus, it is recommended that all women capable of becoming pregnant consume 400 μg from supplements or fortified foods in addition to intake of food folate from a varied diet.

Source: Food and Nutrition Board, National Academy of Sciences.

cont. p. 171

Life stage group	Iodine (µg/d)	Iron (mg/d)	Magnesium (mg/d)	Manganese (mg/d)	Molybdenum (µg/d)	Phosphorus (mg/d)	Selenium (µg/d)	Zinc (mg/d)
Infants								
0–6 mth	110	0.27	30	0.003	2	100	15	2
7–12 mth	130	11	75	0.6	3	275	20	3
Children								
1–3 yr	90	7	80	1.2	17	460	20	3
4–8 yr	90	10	130	1.5	22	500	30	5
Males								
9–13 yr	120	8	240	1.9	34	1,250	40	8
14–18 yr	150	11	410	2.2	43	1,250	55	11
19–30 yr	150	8	400	2.3	45	700	55	11
31–50 yr	150	8	420	2.3	45	700	55	11
51–70 yr	150	8	420	2.3	45	700	55	11
>70 yr	150	8	420	2.3	45	700	55	11
Females								
9–13 yr	120	8	240	1.6	34	1,250	40	8
14–18 yr	150	15	360	1.6	43	1,250	55	9
19–30 yr	150	18	310	1.8	45	700	55	8
31–50 yr	150	18	320	1.8	45	700	55	8
51–70 yr	150	8	320	1.8	45	700	55	8
>70 yr	150	8	320	1.8	45	700	55	8
Pregnancy								
≤18 yr	220	27	400	2.0	50	1,250	60	13
19–30 yr	220	27	350	2.0	50	700	60	11
31–50 yr	220	27	360	2.0	50	700	60	11
Lactation								
≤18 yr	290	10	360	2.6	50	1,250	70	14
19–30 yr	290	9	310	2.6	50	700	70	12
31–50 yr	290	9	320	2.6	50	700	70	12

Appendix B

Chapter Test Answers

Chapter 1

1. F 2. F 3. T 4. F 5. T 6. b 7. b 8. a 9. c
10. d
11. Cells have the ability to make large quantities of cholesterol, so it is not an essential component of the diet.
12. Trace minerals are usually needed in extremely small amounts in the body and, consequently, the diet. Current laboratory methods are generally not sensitive enough to measure minerals in such small quantities. Determining their function in the body is even more difficult.
13. Vitamins regulate a number of important chemical reactions in the body. Although they provide no energy, they help regulate energy metabolism. Vitamins promote cellular growth and reproduction, and their absence in the diet results in specific deficiency diseases.
14. Chronic diseases are long term in nature, they generally develop in response to many factors (not just diet), and there is usually no immediate cure. Although some dietary factors are linked to cancer, family history of cancer plays an important role.
15. Any substance in food that the body assimilates and uses in its metabolic processes can be considered a nutrient. Some nutrients are made in the body in amounts that satisfy requirements, so these nutrients are not considered essential for normal growth and development. Cholesterol is an example of a nutrient that is not needed in the diet, and strict vegetarians who consume no animal products—and therefore no cholesterol—can easily maintain good health. Cholesterol can still be considered a nutrient because when it is consumed, it merges with cholesterol made in the body and is used for a variety of important functions. Other examples of "nonessential" nutrients include the many chemicals found in plants, such as phytosterols and isoflavones, that seem to have a positive impact on overall health by reducing the risk of cancer and other chronic disease, yet they are not required in the diet for growth and development. It is likely that many more nonessential nutrients that improve health and well being will be discovered in the future.

Chapter 2

1. T 2. F 3. F 4. T 5. F 6. c 7. b 8. c 9. a
10. d
11. Because the electrolyte minerals (sodium, potassium, and chloride) easily dissolve in body fluids, they are most likely the major minerals lost through sweat. These minerals can be easily incorporated into sports drinks.
12. In general, the fat-soluble vitamins would be most toxic because they can accumulate in body tissues, particularly the liver, causing metabolic disorders. Excess water-soluble vitamins not used by the body are eliminated via the urine.
13. A milk chocolate candy bar would contain milk and sucrose. The milk contains lactose and would thus provide galactose and glucose. The sucrose would yield glucose and fructose.
14. Dietary fiber is a complex carbohydrate (polysaccharide) and refers to all indigestible plant material consumed by humans. Dietary fiber can be soluble or insoluble in water, but in both cases it passes through the digestive tract without being broken down and absorbed by the body.
15. Trans fatty acids are unsaturated, meaning they contain double bonds. In contrast to cis unsaturated fatty acids, the hydrogen atoms in trans fatty acids are on both sides of the double bond, causing the molecule to have a linear

configuration. Trans fatty acids are found naturally in plant and animal foods, but the primary source of trans fatty acids in the US food supply is hydrogenated vegetable oils. Their impact on health is mediated mainly through their influence on blood cholesterol levels. Trans fatty acids raise blood cholesterol compared to cis unsaturated fatty acids, but lower blood cholesterol when substituted for saturated fatty acids in the diet. There does not appear to be anything uniquely damaging about trans fatty acids to human health and no cases of toxicity have been reported. Trans fatty acids are safe when consumed as part of a well-balanced diet.

Chapter 3

1. T 2. F 3. F 4. T 5. T 6. c 7. a 8. b 9. a
10. d
11. Anaerobic metabolism—and lactic acid production—increases in cells when there is insufficient oxygen for aerobic metabolism. A sedentary person who is "out of shape" probably has a limited capacity to carry enough oxygen in the bloodstream to keep up with the demand for nutrient oxidation via the TCA cycle.
12. Hydrogen atoms are shuttled from plants to animals as components of organic molecules, primarily the macronutrients. Hydrogen is transferred back to plants primarily as a component of water molecules.
13. ATP is a molecule in cells that has the ability to receive energy from dietary macronutrients and transfer that energy directly to metabolic processes in the body.
14. The TCA cycle is a series of chemical reactions in cells that completely oxidizes (or "burns") the macronutrients to CO_2 and H_2O, thus releasing their energy. It is the central component of aerobic metabolism.
15. Plants are able to capture energy from the sun by a process called photosynthesis. Within plant cells, carbon dioxide (CO_2) from the atmosphere is combined with water (H_2O) from the soil to form carbohydrates and, to a lesser extent, lipids and proteins. A byproduct of photosynthesis is oxygen (O_2), which is released into the atmosphere and used by humans and other animals during metabolism of the macronutrients. The overall chemical reaction of photosynthesis can be written as: $CO_2 + H_2O +$ Light Energy $\rightarrow$ Carbohydrate $+ O_2$. In this way, solar energy is captured within the chemical bonds of the macronutrients. Humans obtain these nutrients by consuming plant foods or by consuming animals that have eaten the plants. The nutrients are then broken down by the body so that the energy can be released for cellular functions. The complete breakdown of macronutrients requires oxygen (called metabolic respiration or oxidation) and produces CO_2 and H_2O as byproducts to be recycled back into the environment. The overall breakdown of carbohydrate during energy metabolism is the reverse of photosynthesis and can be written as: Carbohydrate $+ O_2 \rightarrow CO_2 + H_2O +$ Energy. Proteins and triglycerides are also oxidized to $CO_2 + H_2O$ to release their energy. Human cells lack the ability to use energy directly from macronutrients, so the energy is first transferred to an intermediate molecule called adenosine triphosphate (ATP). Cells can use ATP directly in metabolic process that require energy.

Chapter 4

1. T 2. F 3. T 4. F 5. F 6. c 7. d 8. a 9. b
10. c
11. (i) Aim for Fitness, which emphasizes body weight and physical activity; (ii) Build a Healthy Base, which focuses on the Food Guide Pyramid and food safety; and (iii) Choose Sensibly, which emphasizes foods we should consume in low or moderate amounts.
12. Inequitable distribution of food worldwide (due to lack of financial and physical resources and overpopulation) is the primary cause of chronic food shortages. Short-term food shortages can be caused by natural disasters and human-induced events such as war.
13. The average American adult consumes twice the amount of protein needed to meet the body's requirement. In general, availability and consumption of high-protein foods is quite high in affluent societies. Therefore, protein supplements are unnecessary and will not promote muscle growth or performance.
14. In both cases, supplemental nutrient delivery is needed for survival because the patient is unable to eat or digest food. Enteral feeding is preferred because the structure and function

of the gastrointestinal tract is preserved. In some cases, however, parenteral feeding is necessary.

15. Dietary standards represent the specific daily amount of essential nutrients that should be consumed to prevent deficiencies, whereas dietary guidelines are more general in nature and are meant to reduce the risk of chronic diseases such as cancer, osteoporosis, and coronary heart disease. Dietary standards used in the United States were first published in 1943 and are called the Dietary Recommended Allowances (RDAs). The RDAs are based on both scientific research and expert opinion about how much of an essential nutrient is required to prevent deficiencies, but they are set sufficiently high enough to apply to practically all healthy people living in the United States. Dietary guidelines, however, represent advice for the public that is based on social concerns in addition to scientific evidence. The Dietary Guidelines for Americans, published jointly by the US Department of Agriculture and the Department of Health and Human Services, provide the basis for Federal nutrition policy and nutrition education activities. Considerable effort is going into the development of recommendations that incorporate both dietary standards and dietary guidelines. The new Dietary Reference Intakes (DRIs) are based on the old RDAs but will be formulated based on scientific evidence linking specific nutrients to chronic diseases.

Chapter 5

1. F 2. F 3. F 4. T 5. T 6. c 7. d 8. b 9. d
10. a
11. The outside of corn kernels is resistant to enzymatic breakdown in the GI tract. By definition, any plant material that passes through the GI tract undigested is classified as dietary fiber. The kernel's inside, however, is mostly starch and is completely digested and absorbed.
12. Because fructose is absorbed by facilitated diffusion, the amount of fructose on both sides of the intestinal cell membrane will reach equilibrium. The amount inside the cell cannot exceed the amount remaining in the lumen of the small intestine. Bioavailability of fructose is always less than 100%.

13. The constant mixing action of the stomach coupled with peristalsis propels anything ingested through the GI tract.
14. The gallbladder simply stores bile made by the liver. Removal of the gallbladder is meant to open a channel for bile flow into the small intestine. The surgery does not interfere with bile production by the liver.
15. The cookie is physically broken into smaller pieces by mastication in the mouth. The salivary glands release saliva into the mouth that helps to soften and lubricate the cookie. Saliva also contains two enzymes, salivary amylase and lingual lipase, that begin the chemical breakdown of starch and triglyceride, respectively. When the cookie mass is swallowed, it moves into the esophagus and is propelled downward by peristalsis. The gastroesophageal sphincter opens briefly to allow the cookie mass to move into the stomach. Digestive juices in the stomach contain hydrochloric acid and the enzyme pepsin, which initiate the breakdown of protein. After considerable mixing, the cookie mass—now called chyme—is slowly released into the small intestine by rhythmic opening and closing of the pyloric sphincter. The stomach acid is quickly neutralized by bicarbonate produced in the pancreas and released into the small intestine. The pancreatic enzymes trypsin and chymotrypsin continue the chemical breakdown of peptides into amino acids, which can now be absorbed into the intestinal cell. Pancreatic amylase continues the breakdown of starch into the disaccharide maltose. Three enzymes made by the small intestine—maltase, sucrase, and lactase—break down their respective disaccharides into glucose, fructose, and galactose. Only the monosaccharides will be absorbed into the intestinal cell. With the help of bile from the gallbladder, pancreatic lipase breaks down triglyceride into fatty acids and monoglycerides. The dietary lipids must form micelles before they can be absorbed. Vitamins and minerals pass unaltered into the small intestine and are absorbed intact.

Chapter 6

1. T 2. F 3. F 4. F 5. T 6. d 7. b 8. b 9. c
10. b
11. Eating a fat-containing meal results in the

production of chylomicrons, thus temporarily increasing blood triglyceride levels. A person should avoid food for at least 12 hours to allow chylomicrons to completely clear the blood.

12. Insulin controls the "building" reactions that occur in tissues during the absorptive state. It increases the uptake of glucose and amino acids into cells and promotes the synthesis of glycogen, protein, and fatty acids for triglyceride assembly.

13. Galactose is transported to the liver via the hepatic portal vein where it is completely removed from circulation. Galactose is converted to glucose and therefore has the same metabolic fate as glucose.

14. The first use of amino acids is to replenish proteins that have been degraded since the last meal. The liver and muscle require the majority of amino acids for protein synthesis.

15. After absorption into the intestinal cell, glucose enters the hepatic portal vein for direct transport to the liver. About two-thirds of dietary glucose is retained by the liver, where it is converted to glycogen for storage, broken down for energy, or converted to fatty acids for triglyceride synthesis. The other one-third passes through the liver and enters the general circulation as blood glucose. Once in the blood, glucose can be transported to any tissue in the body. The primary users of blood glucose are the brain (which depends on blood glucose as its sole energy source), muscle (which converts it to glycogen for storage), and adipose (which uses glucose as energy for triglyceride synthesis).

Chapter 7

1. F 2. T 3. T 4. T 5. F 6. c 7. d 8. c 9. d
10. b

11. Ketosis occurs in long-term fasting states and is triggered by a gradual decrease in blood glucose (due to lack of dietary carbohydrate). Consequently, adipose cells release fatty acids into the blood at an increased rate. The liver converts the excess fatty acids to ketone bodies which, in turn, increases the blood ketone body concentration.

12. Insulin promotes the uptake of blood glucose into muscle and adipose, which would deprive the brain of needed glucose in the absence of dietary carbohydrate.

13. Glucagon is a hormone that promotes the production and release of glucose by the liver. Glycogen is a storage form of glucose in liver and muscle. Don't be confused by their similarity in spelling.

14. The short-term fasting state is the postabsorptive period (4–48 hours) following a meal. It is part of the normal eating pattern of most people living in developed countries. The long-term fasting state occurs in starvation or when energy-deficient diets are consumed over long periods of time lasting several days or more.

15. In the absorptive state, dietary "energy" is stored as glycogen in the liver and muscle, and as triglyceride in adipose. Although free amino acids are not stored in the body, muscle protein also represents a potential source of energy. In short-term fasting states (such as between meals or overnight fast), liver glycogen is broken down to glucose and released into blood. Maintaining blood glucose levels is critical for the brain, which relies on glucose as its sole energy source. Muscle glycogen provides energy for muscle activity and is not a source of blood glucose. Fatty acids from adipose provide energy for both liver and muscle, and amino acids from muscle protein may also be used in limited amounts for energy in the liver. In long-term fasting states (such as starvation), liver and muscle glycogen is depleted and the body relies more heavily on fatty acids for energy. Triglyceride in adipose is broken down to fatty acids and released into the blood at an accelerated rate. The liver converts the fatty acids to ketone bodies. When the ketone body concentration in blood becomes sufficiently high, the brain and other tissues can use them for energy. Prolonged ketosis is an undesirable metabolic condition that should be avoided.

Chapter 8

1. F 2. F 3. T 4. T 5. F 6. d 7. c 8. a 9. b
10. a

11. Underwater weighing is based on the fact that fat is less dense than water, whereas lean body mass is more dense than water. Once body weight is obtained on land and under water, these values are put into a mathematical equation that calculates the amount of body fat

relative to lean body mass and is expressed as a percentage.

12. The thermic effect of food refers to the energy needed for the mechanical and chemical digestion food. Energy used for this purpose accounts for 5–10% of total energy expenditure by the body.

13. The two major components of long-term weight management are to avoid dieting and to increase physical activity. Establishing reasonable eating patterns is part of the long-term goal of avoiding the weight loss/weight gain cycle that often occurs with dieting.

14. Body fat serves as an energy reserve, an insulator in maintaining constant body temperature, and as a cushion for internal organs. These functions are compromised with insufficient body fat. As a result, muscle "wasting" can occur because the body must rely on amino acids as a source of energy. Too little body fat is also associated with amenorrhea (absence of menstrual cycle), inability to sustain pregnancy, and a decreased ability of the immune system to ward off infection.

15. I would explain that gradual weight gain in adults is almost always due to accumulation of body fat, and that a BMI of 28 would tend to confirm that. I would then explain that achieving a more healthy weight should be approached as a long-term activity and not something that can be attained successfully with short-term dieting. Most energy-restrictive diet plans do not address the issue of how to maintain a stable weight after the initial weight loss. Furthermore, they focus entirely on energy intake and largely ignore the other side of the energy balance equation—energy expenditure. I would encourage my friend to seek nutrition counseling from a registered dietitian to help him establish reasonable eating habits that provide for a well-balanced diet that does not exceed his body's energy needs. In addition, I would encourage him to find ways of increasing physical activity to increase total energy expenditure, which will also strengthen his cardiovascular system and increase muscle tone. By focusing his attention on healthy eating habits and physical activity, he will become more aware of his lifestyle and the behaviors that allowed fat accumulation to occur in the first place. He could then make the necessary behavior modifications that will most likely result in gradual loss of body fat over the long term.

Chapter 9

1. F 2. F 3. T 4. F 5. T 6. d 7. d 8. b 9. c 10. a

11. Trabecular bone is less dense, honeycomb-like bone that is metabolically more active than cortical bone. When blood calcium levels decrease, trabecular bone will quickly release some of its calcium to the bloodstream, making it more susceptible to osteoporosis.

12. Obesity contributes to diabetes mellitus, hypertension, and elevated serum cholesterol levels, thus making it an important risk factor for CHD and stroke.

13. The body's cells have an extremely efficiency "damage control" system that repairs any DNA alterations that occur under most conditions. However, if the cell's ability to repair DNA is overwhelmed by repeated exposure to a carcinogen, the altered DNA will eventually result in the growth and propagation of transformed cancer cells.

14. Heart attacks occur as a direct result of blood clots that form in the arteries that delivery blood (and oxygen) to the heart muscle. The blood clots form in response to a damaged atherosclerotic plaque. Although plaque can restrict blood flow, a heart attack will not occur until a blood clot forms.

15. While there are many factors that contribute to the development of chronic diseases, they can be categorized into environmental (controllable) and genetic (uncontrollable) risk factors. Gender, ethnic background, aging, and family history of disease are examples of genetic risk factors. Being female increases the risk of osteoporosis, particularly after menopause. Estrogen promotes bone formation, so the risk of osteoporosis increases dramatically after menopause. Aging is a risk factor for coronary heart disease, osteoporosis, and non-insulin-dependent diabetes mellitus. Family history is a strong predictor of chronic disease because of the increased chance of inheriting genes that promote disease. Although we have no control over these genetic factors, scientists are currently working on "gene therapies" that could one day help regulate the influence of genes on disease development. In contrast to genetic factors, we do have control over what foods we eat, how much exercise we get, and whether we use tobacco.

Smoking is a strong risk factor for coronary heart disease and certain types of cancer, particularly lung cancer. Diet and physical activity contribute to chronic disease to the extent that they both are part of the energy balance equation and therefore influence body fat, which, in turn, directly impacts coronary heart disease and diabetes mellitus. While both genetic and environmental factors can contribute to chronic disease development, it is impossible to know which factor (or factors) is most important in every individual. Therefore, blanket recommendations regarding controllable risk factors are made with whole populations in mind, with the hope that at least some people will reduce their risk for certain diseases.

Chapter 10

1. F 2. T 3. F 4. T 5. F 6. b 7. a 8. d 9. d
10. c
11. Alcohol, megadoses of vitamins, herbal teas and supplements, and drugs of all type should be avoided during pregnancy. Some experts also recommend avoidance of caffeine.
12. Standard infant formulas are made from cows' milk, which provides protein (whey and casein), carbohydrate (lactose), and some vitamins and minerals. Soy formulas contain soy protein, and sucrose and/or corn syrup as the carbohydrate source. Both types of formula contain added vegetable oils, vitamins, and minerals.
13. Eating breakfast, more fruits and vegetables, and less saturated fat are associated with longevity. People who live longer also "diet" less often, they have fewer fluctuations in body weight, and they tend to remain physically, mentally, and socially active throughout adulthood.
14. The let-down reflex refers to the release of breast milk from the storage lobes to the nipple. The process is controlled by the hormone oxytocin and is stimulated by suckling. Hearing the cries of an infant or simply thinking about breast-feeding can also stimulate the let-down reflex.
15. The life cycle represents a continuum of changing nutritional needs. Nutrition professionals like to define the most obvious stages of change associated with pregnant women, lactating women, infants, young children, teenagers, young adults, and older adults. Pregnant women generally require greater amounts of certain nutrients, particularly iron, folate, and vitamin B_6. Total energy needs also increase about 300 kilocalories per day during the second and third trimesters when fetal growth is greatest. Nutrient requirements for lactating women are also increased above those for non-lactating women and focus mainly on vitamin C, vitamin B_6, and riboflavin. Infants require enough total energy and essential nutrients to support the rapid growth of new tissues. Assuming that a lactating mother is receiving adequate nutrition, breast milk is the ideal food for a growth infant. Commercial formulas can also meet nutrient needs, but they lack a number of other substances, such as immune factors and hormones, that help ensure infant health. A second growth spurt occurs after the onset of puberty and continues until about 16–18 years of age. A healthful diet for children, teenagers, and adults can be based on the Food Guide Pyramid, although portion size will vary with the stage of growth. Specific food selection may also vary with ethnic group. Older adults generally require less total energy because of decreasing physical activity. However, the diet of older adults is often deficient in energy needed to maintain body functions. Many older adults consume diets that contain below the recommended amount of folate, vitamin D, vitamin E, calcium, magnesium, zinc, and water.

Chapter 11

1. F 2. F 3. T 4. T 5. F 6. d 7. b 8. c 9. a
10. d
11. Any abnormal eating behavior could potentially qualify as an eating disorder. However, the term "eating disorder" is generally reserved for abnormal eating behaviors that cause bodily harm and can be diagnosed according to established clinical criteria.
12. Some practical considerations affecting food choice include food availability, cost, and convenience. Access to food may be limited due to inability to shop or physical impairment. The type of foods may be limited to what's being offered at school or the workplace.
13. Obesity can result from overeating (i.e., energy imbalance). People who overeat tend to do so in

response to appetite, not hunger. Individuals can teach themselves to stop eating when they are full by knowing the difference between appetite and hunger and learning to listen to the body's hunger (and satiety) cues.

14. Satiety is the opposite of hunger. It is the feeling of fullness and satisfaction that comes after eating a meal. Satiety is controlled by internal body mechanisms.

15. Most eating disorders are related to body weight or body image. Western societies, such as in the United States, have created a "desirable" body image through the movies, television, and magazines. That image for females is tall and overly thin, while the image for males is lean and overly muscular. While few people in society are able to achieve such an appearance, the desire to look this way can be overwhelming. Pressure from friends or family to look and act a certain way can further compound the problem. Other pressures such as achieving good grades, holding down a job, or having responsibilities at home can impact a person's self-esteem, which can also contribute to eating disorders. All of these external influences can directly or indirectly cause people to develop distorted views of food, healthful eating habits, and their bodies.

Chapter 12

1. T 2. F 3. F 4. T 5. F 6. c 7. d 8. b 9. a 10. d

11. The Dietary Guidelines for Americans contain nutrition information based on scientific research and expert review of the evidence. The Guidelines are published by the US Department of Agriculture and the Department of Health and Human Services. Nutrition and health information distributed in magazines, newspapers, infomercials, and television and radio reports are all financially driven and are therefore prone to fraudulent or misleading health claims aimed at capturing attention and boosting sales.

12. Gathering the results of each research study is like creating one piece of a complicated jigsaw puzzle. Developing an understanding of the picture occurs only after a significant number of puzzle pieces are assembled. Careful judgment should be used when speculating about the picture when too many pieces are missing.

13. When an exposure and an outcome occur together in an obvious pattern they are said to be "associated." Such an association, however, provides no information about whether the exposure causes the outcome.

14. A hypothesis is an assumption that is made to explain an observation. As part of the scientific method, hypotheses are tested with experimentation and either accepted or rejected based on the study's results.

15. When judging the headline, the first keyword is "risk." This suggests that an association was discovered between the consumption of high-fat diets and the occurrence of breast cancer. This also suggests that a study (or studies) was conducted. Even without the full article, these aspects can be inferred from the headline. Therefore, the best place to start would be to understand as thoroughly as possible the nature of the study, including study design, the hypothesis being tested, how fat intake and breast cancer were measured, etc. If this turns out to be a legitimate scientific study, then the results should be compared to other studies that examined fat intake with breast cancer to see how the current study fits into the larger picture ("Does this study make sense?"). It is also important to know if the researchers had a vested interest in seeing an association between dietary fat and breast cancer ("Do they stand to profit from the results?"). Newspaper articles usually include statements made by the researchers or other interested parties that are intended to increase excitement for the reader; therefore, judging these unconfirmed comments against the study's results will be necessary. Finally, making a list of all the unanswered questions will help evaluate how this newspaper article has contributed to (or detracted from) our overall understanding of how diet is related to breast cancer.

Chapter 13

1. T 2. F 3. T 4. F 5. T 6. b 7. c 8. a 9. c 10. d

11. Food-borne infection is an illness caused by the ingestion of relatively large numbers of pathogenic bacteria. Food-borne intoxication is an illness caused by the ingestion of a toxin. Most

cases of food-borne intoxication are caused by consuming toxin-producing bacteria, although ingestion of nonbacterial toxins can also cause illness.

12. The primary reason for food labels is to provide consumers with detailed information about the nutrient content of food products. Food labels are designed to help consumers make food purchasing decisions and to plan their diets wisely.

13. A functional food is a manufactured product in which an ingredient has been added that is not normally associated with that product. It is believed that the added substance will provide health benefits beyond the basic nutrient requirements of the body.

14. Calcium-fortified orange juice; vitamin D-fortified milk; iodine-fortified table salt; folic acid-fortified pasta; iron-fortified breakfast cereal; vitamin C-fortified grape juice (and other fruit juices naturally low in vitamin C).

15. The primary goals of the food processing industry are to make food safer and to minimize spoilage. These goals are achieved through methods that inhibit the growth of the microorganisms that cause spoilage and illness when consumed. Ways in which foods are processed include treatment with temperature, the use of food additives, and various packaging techniques. These processing methods also improve the quality of foods by enhancing their color, flavor, and texture thus making them more appealing to the consumer. Virtually every food we consume is processed in some way. Even a head of lettuce is harvested, cleaned and trimmed, wrapped in plastic, transported to a produce wholesaler, and finally shipped to the grocery store. Other types of food products may require more elaborate processing techniques. Some people have questioned the safety of food additives, although most are natural substances found in nature. Compared to the benefits they provide, the risk of using food additives is quite small. The food supply in the United States is one of the safest, most wholesome in the world, largely due to modern food processing techniques.

Chapter 14

1. F 2. T 3. F 4. T 5. F 6. b 7. c 8. d 9. a
10. d

11. Fitness is a term that describes how well an individual can perform physical activity. Someone who is physically fit has an increased capacity to deliver oxygen to muscle cells for use in the oxidation of the macronutrients.

12. Good health is often defined as a person's state of well being in the absence of disease. Optimal health can be thought of as being at the maximum upper end of the "good health" spectrum.

13. Registered dietitians are food and nutrition professionals who have fulfilled the requirements established by the American Dietetic Association. Their education and training include a minimum of a bachelor's degree (with specific coursework requirements), completion of a supervised practice program (internship), and they must pass the national registration examination.

14. Regular exercise reduces the risk of heart disease, osteoporosis, and some types of cancer. Exercise reduces the risk of obesity and related conditions, such as diabetes mellitus and hypertension. People who exercise also claim to have reduced stress and anxiety, as well as improved sleeping and mental function. Exercise strengthens the heart muscle and improves the oxygen-carrying capacity of the cardiovascular system.

15. Aerobic metabolism is the breakdown of macronutrients *in the presence of oxygen* for release of energy. Aerobic metabolism is the most efficient way to provide energy to muscle.

Appendix C

Topic Tests

Chapter 1

Topic Test 1.1: The Many Faces of Nutrition

True/False

1. A complete understanding of nutrition encompasses the social, psychological, economic, and spiritual aspects of food and health.
2. "Nutrition" may be defined as "the interactions between food and living organisms."

Multiple Choice

3. Which of the follow careers are related to nutrition?
   a. Food scientist
   b. Dietitian
   c. Psychologist
   d. All of the above
4. Dr. James Lind of the Royal British Navy is generally credited with what?
   a. Discovering a cure for scurvy
   b. Conducting one of the first controlled research studies in nutrition
   c. Demonstrating a link between specific foods and deficiency diseases
   d. All of the above

Review Questions

5. What courses would you expect to find in a university nutrition program?
6. Identify some careers that require an appreciation of basic nutrition principles.

Topic Test 1.2: Evolution of Nutrition Science

True/False

1. All of the essential nutrients have been discovered and are well documented.

2. Philosophers in ancient China first proposed the concept that a specific substance in food could prevent a specific disease.

Multiple Choice

3. Some of the first experiments aimed at recreating a food product in the laboratory involved
   a. Honey
   b. Milk
   c. Lemon juice
   d. Egg yolks
4. Why do you suppose British sailors are nicknamed "limeys"?
   a. Their navy guns used to fire cannonballs the size of limes
   b. British sailors were once paid with limes and other citrus fruit
   c. Scurvy was a common disease among sailors, which caused their skin to turn green
   d. British sailors consumed lime juice on long voyages to prevent scurvy

Review Questions

5. What is a nutrient deficiency disease?
6. What is a chronic disease?

Topic Test 1.3: Definition of a Nutrient

True/False

1. Nutrients and drugs can sometimes cause the same metabolic responses.
2. Some nutrients can become "essential" if the body stops producing them in amounts large enough to meet the body's needs.

Multiple Choice

3. Which health organization is responsible for publishing the official definition of a nutrient?
   a. American Medical Association
   b. American Society for Nutritional Sciences

c. American Dietetic Association
d. None of the above
4. Essential nutrients
   a. Are found only in milk and dairy products
   b. Can be made by the body in adequate amounts
   c. Are required for normal growth, development, and maintenance of health
   d. All of the above

Review Questions

5. Describe the difference between "essential" and "nonessential" nutrients?
6. What was the classic definition of a nutrient?

Topic Test 1.4: Overview of the Nutrient Classes

True/False

1. Dietary proteins are found exclusively in meat, poultry, and other animal products.
2. Triglycerides are found throughout the food supply in both plant and animal products.

Multiple Choice

3. Which is the most abundant nutrient class in the human diet?
   a. Carbohydrates
   b. Minerals
   c. Water
   d. Lipids
4. Which of the following is not considered a carbohydrate?
   a. Cholesterol
   b. Fiber
   c. Sugar
   d. Starch

Review Questions

5. What is the difference between a "fat" and an "oil"?
6. Describe the macronutrients.

Topic Test 1.1: Answers

1. **True.** The broad scope of nutrition makes it a truly multidisciplinary field of study.
2. **True.** While other definitions could be formulated, the most useful definition should be broad enough to encompass all of the many aspects and perspectives that contribute to nutrition.
3. **d.** The field of nutrition involves many types of careers that, at some level, are concerned with food, diet, and health (both physical and psychological health).
4. **d.** Although food had been used for centuries to treat ill health, Lind is thought to be the first scientist to establish a clear relationship between a specific deficiency disease and the lack of a specific nutrient.
5. Most 4-year programs in nutrition require courses related to the human body, such as physiology, anatomy, cell biology, chemistry, and biochemistry. Courses related to food would include food chemistry, commercial food production, food preparation and foodservice management, and global and cultural aspects of foods. Most nutrition programs also include courses in clinical and community nutrition, which emphasize nutrition education and counseling.
6. Careers that require an understanding of nutrition principles include dietetics, food industry, pharmacy, dentistry, medicine, epidemiology, public health, and psychology when the emphasis is on nutrition counseling and abnormal eating patterns.

Topic Test 1.2: Answers

1. **False.** Other essential nutrients may yet be discovered as laboratory methods become more sensitive and our understanding of nutrition increases. Choline is an example of a nutrient that, until now, was not considered to be essential.
2. **False.** The concept was first suggested by Lind about 250 years ago, and gained wide acceptance during the past century.
3. **b.** Several researchers in the late nineteenth century attempted to reproduce milk as a substitute formula for breast-feeding.
4. **d.** The British physician Lind was the first to treat a dietary deficiency disease (scurvy) with a specific food (lime and lemon juice).
5. Any disease or abnormal condition that develops when an essential nutrient is absent from the diet or consumed in amounts too low to meet the body's requirement for normal function. Scurvy is an example of a clinical disease that develops when inadequate amounts of vitamin C are consumed.
6. Chronic diseases are generally long-term debilitating diseases such as cancer, osteoporosis, and heart disease. Unlike specific deficiency diseases, chronic diseases may have many causes of which diet is only one contributing factor.

Topic Test 1.3: Answers

1. **True.** Both nutrients and drugs have the ability to treat, cure, and prevent disease, usually by the same metabolic processes.
2. **True.** A person may require certain nutrients in the diet if normal body function is compromised because of illness.
3. **d.** Because nutrients have such a broad role in health and disease, and because our knowledge about nutrients continues to evolve, these health organization are reluctant to publish official definitions.
4. **c.** The absence of a single essential nutrient in the diet will result in impaired growth or a specific deficiency symptom.
5. An essential nutrient must be consumed in the diet because the body does not make it, or makes it in amounts too low to meet the body's needs. A nonessential nutrient can be made in the body in adequate amounts and is therefore not required in the diet. However, the body still has the ability to use nonessential nutrients if they are consumed.
6. Chemical substances required in the diet for normal growth, development, and maintenance of health.

Topic Test 1.4: Answers

1. **False.** Several plant foods such as soybeans, lentils, and nuts are rich sources of dietary protein.
2. **True.** Both animal fats and vegetable oils are basically 100% triglyceride.
3. **c.** In addition to being the most abundant dietary nutrient, water is the major component of the human body.
4. **a.** Cholesterol does not dissolve in water and is considered a lipid.
5. Fats and oils belong to the same chemical family called triglycerides. They are essentially the same thing, except that fats are solid at room temperature while oils are liquid. All triglycerides are considered lipids because they do not dissolve in water.
6. Carbohydrates, proteins, and lipids are considered macronutrients because they are needed in the diet in relatively large amounts. Unlike vitamins, minerals and water, the macronutrients provide the body with energy.

Chapter 2

Topic Test 2.1: Carbohydrates
True/False
1. Carbohydrates are the most widely consumed macronutrients in the world.
2. macroSoluble fiber is different than insoluble fiber because it is partially digested in the gastrointestinal tract of humans.

Multiple Choice
3. Which of the following is not considered a "sugar"?
   a. Glucose
   b. Amylose
   c. Maltose
   d. Lactose
4. The most abundant carbohydrate consumed by humans is
   a. Sucrose
   b. Lactose
   c. Fructose
   d. Glucose

Review Questions
5. Explain why high-fructose corn syrups are used extensively in the food industry.
6. Describe the chemical structure of starch.

Topic Test 2.2: Proteins
True/False
1. There are over 100 amino acids used in protein synthesis, which allows the body to make several thousand different types of proteins.
2. Dietary proteins are found only in animal foods.

Multiple Choice
3. Which of the following substances found in the body are proteins?
   a. Enzymes
   b. Antibodies
   c. Hormones
   d. All of the above
4. A type of protein deficiency called kwashiorkor has which of the following symptoms?
   a. Severe muscle wasting
   b. Bloated abdomen
   c. Loss of hair
   d. Swollen tongue

Review Questions
5. What is the difference between essential and nonessential amino acids?
6. What is a limiting amino acid?

Topic Test 2.3: Lipids
True/False
1. Dietary fats (triglycerides) are readily available in developed countries, but are not essential nutrients in the human diet.
2. Cholesterol is a vitally important substance in the body, but it is not required in the diet.

Multiple Choice
3. Two fatty acids attached to glycerol is called a
   a. Monoglyceride
   b. Diglyceride
   c. Triglyceride
   d. Transglyceride
4. The term "omega-3" refers to a fatty acid that
   a. Has three glycerol molecules attached to it
   b. Has three hydrogen atoms attached to it
   c. Has three double bonds
   d. Has a double bond three carbons from the end

Review Questions
5. What is meant by fatty acid "saturation"?
6. Where are trans fatty acids found in the food supply?

Topic Test 2.4: Vitamins
True/False
1. Choline is a recently discovered vitamin.
2. The B-complex vitamins are usually bound together in foods forming large complexes.

Multiple Choice
3. What is the primary function of vitamins?
   a. Regulate chemical reactions in the body
   b. Provide energy
   c. Transport nutrients in the blood
   d. Act as structural components of cells
4. Which vitamin is likely to be toxic if consumed in excess amount for a long period of time?
   a. Vitamin C
   b. Vitamin B_{12}
   c. Riboflavin
   d. Vitamin A

Review Questions
5. What are phytochemicals?
6. What are bogus vitamins?

Topic Test 2.5: Minerals
True/False
1. Electrolytes are essential minerals that dissolve in body fluids and conduct electricity.
2. Not all minerals are essential nutrients, because the body can make certain minerals.

Multiple Choice
3. What two minerals comprise the main structural component of bone?
   a. Sodium and phosphorus
   b. Sodium and potassium
   c. Calcium and phosphorus
   d. Calcium and chloride
4. How are the major minerals different from the trace minerals?
   a. Major minerals are found in greater amounts in the body
   b. Major minerals perform more important functions than trace minerals
   c. Major minerals are larger molecules than trace minerals
   d. All of the above

Review Questions
5. How does iron deficiency result in anemia?
6. Why is it not necessary for everyone to limit their sodium intake?

Topic Test 2.6: Water
True/False
1. About one-third of the water consumed by adults comes from food, not beverages.
2. Bottled water is usually safer and healthier than municipal water supplies.

Multiple Choice
3. Which of the following is **not** a common cause of dehydration?
   a. Diarrhea
   b. Consumption of coffee
   c. Consumption of sports drinks
   d. Strenuous exercise
4. What minimum percentage of body water lost will result in dehydration?
   a. 20%
   b. 10%
   c. 5%
   d. 2%

Review Questions
5. Describe water balance.

6. Explain why someone on a high-protein diet should increase his or her water consumption.

Topic Test 2.1: Answers

1. **True.** High-starch foods form the dietary base for most populations throughout the world.
2. **False.** The term "soluble" fiber simply means it dissolves in water, but it is still not digested by humans.
3. **b.** Amylose is a type of starch and therefore a complex carbohydrate (polysaccharide). All mono- and disaccharides are simple carbohydrates (sugars).
4. **d.** Because glucose comprises part of sucrose and lactose, and is the only monosaccharide in starch, it is by far the most abundant carbohydrate in the food supply.
5. Of all the simple carbohydrates, fructose is the sweetest tasting. Therefore, high fructose corn syrups can replace sucrose in many food products as the primary sweetening agent. Less high fructose corn syrup is needed and it is currently less expensive than sucrose.
6. Starch contains long chains of the monosaccharide glucose. It may exist as a single chain (amylose) or it may have several branched chains (amylopectin). Most plant starch contains both types, but amylopectin usually comprises about 75% of the total starch.

Topic Test 2.2: Answers

1. **False.** There are only 20 amino acids used by humans for protein synthesis; nine are essential and 11 are nonessential. The body still makes thousands of different proteins from just 20 amino acids.
2. **False.** Proteins are found in both plant and animal foods. Dietary protein from both sources is generally more abundant in developed countries.
3. **d.** All of the body's enzymes and antibodies are proteins. Some hormones are proteins, although some hormones are made from other molecules besides protein.
4. **b.** Kwashiorkor occurs when diets are adequate in total energy, but deficient in protein. This causes fluid accumulation in the abdomen, resulting in bloated bellies.
5. Both essential and nonessential amino acids are required for protein synthesis. However, humans cannot make the essential amino acids and must consume them in the diet. Nonessential amino acids are made in the body.

6. Every protein in the human body has a specific number and sequence of amino acids in its chemical structure. If just one amino acid is in short supply, the protein cannot be synthesized in large enough quantities to meet requirements. The essential amino acid that is available in the lowest amount is called the limiting amino acid.

Topic Test 2.3: Answers

1. **False.** Linoleic acid and linolenic acid are essential for growth and maintenance of health. The source of these two fatty acids is dietary triglyceride.
2. **True.** Cholesterol functions in virtually every cell in the body, but adequate amounts can be made within the cell.
3. **b.** Monoglycerides have one fatty acid attached to glycerol, diglycerides have two fatty acids, and triglycerides have three.
4. **d.** The omega system describes the position of the last double bond in the fatty acid carbon chain.
5. A fatty acid is "saturated" with hydrogen atoms when no double bonds exist in the molecule. Inclusion of one double bond yields a monounsaturated fatty acid; two or more double bonds yields a polyunsaturated fatty acid. The degree of saturation is directly related to how solid the fatty acid is at room temperature.
6. Trans fatty acids are found naturally in the fat of ruminant animals, such as milk fat and beef tallow. Some plant foods also contain trans fatty acids, but usually in very low concentrations. Most trans fatty acids consumed by humans come from hydrogenated vegetable oils.

Topic Test 2.4: Answers

1. **Not exactly.** Choline was discovered many years ago to have an important function in the body. It only recently has been suggested that the body does not make enough choline to meet requirements and, therefore, it should be recognized as an essential nutrient and given vitamin status.
2. **False.** Use of the term "complex" is unfortunate because the B vitamins are not bound together. They exist independently in foods.
3. **a.** Vitamins do not contain energy, nor do they function as transporters or structural components of cells.
4. **d.** Because vitamin A is fat soluble, it can easily accumulate to toxic levels in body tissues, particularly the liver. The other vitamins are water

soluble and therefore excreted in the urine if not used by the body.

5. Phytochemicals are substances in plants that may have beneficial properties in reducing the risk of certain diseases and metabolic disorders. Phytochemicals are not considered essential nutrients because their absence in the diet does not produce specific deficiency diseases.

6. Bogus vitamins are substances sold as essential nutrients, but they are not required in the diet and their absence does not produce deficiency diseases. In some cases, the substances are not normally found in the body and perform no specific function.

Topic Test 2.5: Answers

1. True. Electrolytes participate in important electrochemical and electromechanical functions, such as nerve impulses and muscle contraction.

2. False. Minerals are basic elements of the earth that cannot be created or broken down by the body. Therefore, all minerals required by the body must be obtained from the diet.

3. c. Calcium and phosphorus form a crystalline structure called hydroxyapatite that is the main foundation of bone tissue.

4. a. The major minerals are found in the body in amounts greater than 0.05% total body weight.

5. Iron is a critical component of hemoglobin, which in turn is a component of red blood cells. Oxygen is transported in the bloodstream attached to hemoglobin. When dietary iron is in short supply, neither hemoglobin nor red blood cells will be produced in great enough quantity to meet oxygen demand in the tissues.

6. High sodium intake has been linked to hypertension (high blood pressure). Consequently, health organizations have traditionally advised people with hypertension to limit their sodium intake. However, not every person with hypertension is "salt-sensitive" and such a blanket recommendation may not be necessary for people who do not have hypertension or have no family history of the disease.

Topic Test 2.6: Answers

1. True. About 3–4 cups of water per day are consumed as water-containing foods. Adults need about 10 cups of water per day (food + beverages) to prevent dehydration.

2. False. Bottled water may taste better than tap water, but it is usually no safer or healthier. In fact, 25% of bottled water sold in the US comes from tap water.

3. c. Coffee contains caffeine which increases urinary output, while sports drinks contain no caffeine. Exercise can increase water loss through sweat and increased respiration.

4. d. As little as 2% loss of body water will produce the symptoms of dehydration, including headache and nausea.

5. Water balance refers to the amount of water consumed versus the amount of body water lost every day. Negative water balance can result in dehydration (which is very common), while positive water balance can result in water toxicity (not very common).

6. Excess dietary protein needs extra body water for processing and removal from the body through the kidneys (increased urinary output).

Chapter 3

Topic Test 3.1: Energy—Universal Life Support

True/False

1. Mechanical energy is the only form of energy present in the human body.

2. The main function of photosynthesis is to make carbohydrate from carbon dioxide and water.

Multiple Choice

3. One Calorie, when written with a capital "C," is equal to
   a. 1,000 kilocalories
   b. 1,000 kcal
   c. 1 calorie
   d. 1,000 calories

4. The type of energy inherent in a steam engine is an example of
   a. Mechanical energy
   b. Electrical energy
   c. Heat energy
   d. Light energy

Review Questions

5. Calculate how much energy is in a glass of milk containing 12 grams of carbohydrate, 8 grams of protein, and 5 grams of fat.

6. Why is photosynthesis in plants so important to human nutrition?

Topic Test 3.2: Nutrient Recycling

True/False

1. Consumption of protein is the primary means by which nitrogen is transferred from plants to humans.
2. Plants receive most of their oxygen atoms by uptake from the atmosphere.

Multiple Choice

3. All of the following are examples of organic molecules except
   a. Calcium
   b. Vitamin C
   c. Sucrose
   d. Triglyceride
4. Oxygen atoms can enter the human through each of the following except
   a. Breathing air
   b. Taking a mineral supplement
   c. Drinking milk
   d. Eating red meat

Review Questions

5. How is carbon recycled between plants and animals?
6. Describe how the nitrogen atoms within protein molecules consumed by humans are recycled back into the environment.

Topic Test 3.3: Nutrients as Energy Distributors

True/False

1. Cells require energy only after a meal when the macronutrients are available.
2. Energy can be temporarily stored in the body in the form of glycogen.

Multiple Choice

3. During normal energy metabolism, dietary glucose is converted to pyruvate in a process called
   a. Gluconeosis
   b. Glycolysis
   c. Gluconeogenesis
   d. Glycopyrolysis
4. The tricarboxylic acid (TCA) cycle
   a. Is responsible for transforming most of the food energy used in the body
   b. Oxidizes acetyl-CoA to CO_2 and H_2O
   c. Produces ATP molecules
   d. All of the above

Review Questions

5. Describe the function of ATP.
6. What is the significance of pyruvate in macronutrient metabolism?

Topic Test 3.1: Answers

1. **False.** Examples of all forms of energy are found in the human body. For example, light energy performs work in the eye, electrical energy is needed for proper nerve function, and heat energy helps regulate body temperature.
2. **True.** Photosynthesis is the only original source of carbohydrate on the planet earth.
3. **d.** One Calorie = 1,000 calories (or 1 kilocalorie)
4. **c.** The primary "work" is generated by heat energy. However, the heat energy must be converted to mechanical energy through gears and levers in order to make the wheels turn.
5. (12 grams carbohydrate $\times$ 4 kcal/g) + (8 grams protein $\times$ 4 kcal/g) + (5 grams fat $\times$ 9 kcal/g) = (48 kcal from carbohydrate) + (32 kcal from protein) + (45 kcal from fat) = 125 total kcalories
6. Humans depend on dietary carbohydrate, protein, and fat as their energy sources. Photosynthesis generates these nutrients in the plants and is responsible for their presence in virtually every biological system and throughout the food supply. Photosynthesis also provides oxygen needed for metabolic processes in animals and other organisms.

Topic Test 3.2: Answers

1. **True.** The vast majority of nitrogen in human diets is in the form of amino acids and proteins. Nitrogen in the soil and air is captured by plants and converted to protein that is eaten directly by grazing animals, which in turn are eaten by humans.
2. **False.** Plants get most of their oxygen atoms from CO_2 in the atmosphere and H_2O in the soil.
3. **a.** Vitamin C, sucrose, and triglycerides are examples of molecules containing carbon atoms. Calcium is a mineral and therefore contains no carbon.
4. **b.** Air contains gaseous oxygen, milk is mostly water (H_2O), and red meat contains several organic molecules that contain oxygen atoms. Minerals contain no oxygen.
5. Carbon is transferred from humans and animals back to plants in the form of CO_2. Through photosynthesis, plants incorporate carbon into organic molecules, which are transferred to

humans in the food supply as carbohydrates, proteins, lipids, and vitamins.

6. After consumption, proteins are eventually metabolized (broken down) in the body. The nitrogen is excreted in urine and feces.

Topic Test 3.3: Answers

1. **False.** Cells need a continuous supply of energy, regardless of one's dietary status.
2. **True.** Dietary carbohydrates, primarily glucose, can be converted to glycogen and stored in the liver and muscle.
3. **b.** Conversion of glucose to pyruvate is called glycolysis; conversion of pyruvate to glucose is called gluconeogenesis.
4. **d.** About two-thirds of all dietary energy is released during the oxidation of acetyl-CoA via the TCA cycle, which results in the transfer of the energy to ATP.
5. The energy in carbohydrate, protein, and triglyceride cannot be extracted and used directly by cells. ATP serves as an acceptor of the energy from dietary macronutrients, then transfers the energy to the cells by actively participating in chemicals reactions.
6. For energy to be released from glucose and some amino acids, these molecules must first be converted to pyruvate. This provides the opportunity for glucose and amino acids to be interconverted, thus shifting the nutrient energy between molecules.

Chapter 4

Topic Test 4.1: Global Food Availability

True/False

1. Current estimates show that economic growth and food production are beginning to lag behind the world's population growth.
2. One of the most common diseases resulting from food shortages is heart disease.

Multiple Choice

3. The leading cause of death among children in developing countries is
   a. Rickets

b. Vitamin A deficiency
c. Dermatitis
d. Diarrhea

4. Famine is almost always the direct result of
   a. Decreased farmland
   b. Crop failure
   c. Increased birth rate
   d. Poverty

Review Questions

5. What is the major cause of food shortages worldwide?
6. Even though there is currently enough food in the world to feed the entire population, food shortages exist. Why?

Topic Test 4.2: Dietary Recommendations

True/False

1. The first dietary recommendations were developed in England in response to the Industrial Revolution.
2. Consumers should select foods from the top of the Food Guide Pyramid most frequently.

Multiple Choice

3. Which of the following is not a major goal of the 2000 Dietary Guidelines for Americans?
   a. Choose sensibly
   b. Eat plentifully
   c. Aim for fitness
   d. Build a healthy base

4. In general, dietary recommendations are intended to
   a. Maximize food efficiency
   b. Increase athletic performance
   c. Increase water consumption
   d. Maintain public health

Review Questions

5. What are dietary standards?
6. Describe the Food Guide Pyramid.

Topic Test 4.3: Dietary Supplements

True/False

1. Protein supplements will help physically active people increase muscle mass.
2. There is no law in the United States regulating the manufacture of dietary supplements.

Multiple Choice

3. Which of the following is not commonly sold as a dietary supplement?
   a. Proteins
   b. Amino acids
   c. Vitamins
   d. Disaccharides
4. Which person is most likely to require a vitamin and/or mineral supplement?
   a. High school male football player
   b. Pregnant female
   c. Forty-year-old male professor
   d. Sixty-year-old female executive

Review Questions

5. Why are supplements containing metabolic chemicals generally safer than herbal supplements?
6. Explain why just because a dietary supplement is made with all natural ingredients, it is not necessarily safe.

Topic Test 4.1: Answers

1. **True.** The rate at which the population is growing shows no signs of slowing in the near future, suggesting that food shortages will continuing to plague many who live in underdeveloped countries.
2. **False.** Heart disease, cancer, hypertension (high blood pressure), and diabetes are diseases generally related to overconsumption of food in developed countries.
3. **d.** Increased susceptibility to infection results in a high incidence of diarrhea among children in developing countries.
4. **b.** Whether from hurricanes, floods, or human foolishness, crop failure is directly responsible for widespread food shortages associated with famine.
5. The primary cause of food shortages is overpopulation in certain regions of the world and the inability to provide enough food for those populations. Food shortages can also be caused by famine, but overpopulation accounts for a greater proportion of disease and death related to food shortages worldwide.
6. Despite having enough food to adequately feed every person on earth, the food supply is not equally distributed around the world. Inequitable distribution and inaccessibility are major factors preventing many populations from receiving the levels of nutrients needed to maintain good health.

Topic Test 4.2: Answers

1. **True.** The British government developed the first dietary recommendations in the mid-1800s as a way to keep their large industrial workforce healthy and productive.
2. **False.** The top of the Food Guide Pyramid represents fats, oil, and sweets. These foods should be used sparingly.
3. **b.** Eating "plentifully" could lead to overconsumption of food and therefore contribute to obesity.
4. **d.** By following dietary recommendations (both standards and guidelines), nutrient deficiencies can be avoided and the risk of chronic diseases may be reduced.
5. Dietary standards are specific amounts of essential nutrients that should be consumed each day to prevent deficiencies. The values for each nutrient are set sufficiently high so that they apply to practically all healthy people within a group or population. The RDAs (and the new DRIs) are the dietary standards used in the United States.
6. The Food Guide Pyramid is intended to help people make healthy food choices when planning an overall diet. It shows six different food groups and the recommended number of servings a person should consume each day for good health. When followed properly, The Food Guide Pyramid will provide all the nutrients needed to prevent deficiency and reduce the risk of chronic disease.

Topic Test 4.3: Answers

1. **False.** The only way to increase muscle mass is to increase the workload of muscle. As long as dietary protein is meeting the body's needs (Americans already consume twice the requirement amount), taking protein supplements will do absolutely nothing except drain your bank account.
2. **True.** The Dietary Supplement Health and Education Act of 1994 requires only that supplements be labeled "dietary supplement" and that the label indicates the recommended serving size and the name and amount of each ingredient per serving.
3. **d.** The most abundant disaccharides in the food supply are sucrose (table sugar) and lactose (milk sugar). They are readily available and consumed in quantities that far exceed those typically found in supplements.

4. **d.** Pregnancy is the only condition listed in which the body's requirement for essential nutrients is increased. Nutrient requirements can often be met through normal diet in the other situations.

5. Metabolic chemicals are normally found in the body, whereas herbal supplements contain chemicals that are foreign to the body. Therefore, herbal supplements are more likely to be toxic at lower doses.

6. The safety of a dietary supplement depends on the type and amount of chemicals ingested, regardless of whether those chemicals are found in nature or made in the laboratory.

Chapter 5

Topic Test 5.1: Digestion
True/False
1. Enzymes are required for complete digestion and absorption of nutrients.
2. Bicarbonate made in the pancreas is released into the small intestine to help digest lipids.

Multiple Choice
3. Food passes through the following sections of the gastrointestinal tract in which order?
    a. Mouth, esophagus, liver, stomach, small intestine, large intestine, rectum
    b. Mouth, esophagus, stomach, liver, small intestine, large intestine, rectum
    c. Mouth, stomach, small intestine, pancreas, large intestine, rectum
    d. Mouth, esophagus, stomach, small intestine, large intestine, rectum
4. The primary function of villi and microvilli is to
    a. Provide a large surface area for nutrient absorption
    b. Propel food through the digestive tract
    c. Produce hydrochloric acid for protein digestion
    d. Store bile until needed for lipid digestion

Review Questions
5. What are the final products of digestion that can be absorbed in the small intestine?
6. How does bile help in lipid digestion?

Topic Test 5.2: Mechanisms of Nutrient Absorption
True/False
1. Absorption refers to the enzymatic breakdown of nutrients within the gastrointestinal tract.
2. Bile acids are made in the liver from cholesterol.

Multiple Choice
3. What mechanism of nutrient absorption requires both a carrier protein and the input of energy?
    a. Active transport
    b. Passive diffusion
    c. Facilitated diffusion
    d. None of the above
4. Bioavailability refers to
    a. How much energy is required to absorb nutrients
    b. The time required for food to be digested
    c. The amount of food available to a population
    d. How efficiently a nutrient is absorbed

Review Questions
5. Describe how micelles are formed.
6. Explain how passive diffusion works?

Topic Test 5.3: Nutrient Destinations
True/False
1. About two-thirds of dietary glucose is retained by the liver when first absorbed.
2. Water-soluble vitamins and minerals consumed in excess of body needs are excreted in the urine.

Multiple Choice
3. Chylomicrons
    a. Are formed in the cells of the small intestine
    b. Enter the lymphatic system prior to transport in the bloodstream
    c. Are made only when a fat-containing meal is consumed
    d. All of the above
4. Which of the following tissues is not a major user of glucose?
    a. Brain
    b. Adipose
    c. Pancreas
    d. Muscle

Review Questions

5. Describe what happens to amino acids after absorption.
6. Explain why fructose and galactose—while absorbed from the diet—are not found in the circulating blood.

Topic Test 5.1: Answers

1. **True.** Enzymes regulate all metabolic processes in the body by controlling the rate of chemical reactions. In digestion, enzymes speed up the breakdown of large nutrients into smaller units that can be absorbed in the small intestine.
2. **False.** The function of bicarbonate is to neutralize the stomach acid that passes into small intestine during normal digestion.
3. **d.** The liver and pancreas are accessory organs; therefore, food does not pass through them. The primary function of accessory organs is to produce digestive juices that are released into the gastrointestinal tract.
4. **a.** Villi and microvilli increase the surface area of the small intestine approximately 1,000 times, thereby increasing the efficiency of nutrient absorption.
5. Carbohydrate digestion yields glucose, fructose, and galactose. Protein digestion yields amino acids. Triglyceride digestion yields fatty acids and monoglycerides.
6. Bile is made in the liver and stored in the gallbladder. When a fat-containing meal is consumed, the gallbladder releases bile into the small intestine where it acts as a detergent by breaking lipid into very small particles. The detergent action helps pancreatic lipase digest triglycerides into fatty acids and monoglycerides.

Topic Test 5.2: Answers

1. **False.** Absorption refers to the movement of nutrients from the lumen of the gastrointestinal tract into the cells that line the surface of the small intestine.
2. **True.** Cholesterol serves as the building block for several important compounds in the body.
3. **a.** Because active transport uses a specific carrier protein and energy input, it can move nutrients across the cell membrane from regions of low nutrient concentration to regions of high concentration. The advantage is that absorption efficiency can be nearly 100%.
4. **d.** Bioavailability of a nutrient is usually expressed as the percent absorbed.
5. The presence of dietary fatty acids and monoglycerides in the small intestine signals the release of bile (containing bile acids and phospholipids) from the gallbladder. The bile acids and phospholipids act as detergents, breaking the dietary lipid into very small droplets that are easily absorbed.
6. Passive diffusion is driven by a "concentration gradient" in which nutrients move through the intestinal cell membrane from the side with highest concentration to the side with lowest concentration. In this way, an equilibrium is reached where the concentration on both sides is approximately equal. The absorption efficiency (bioavailability) will always be less than 100% for nutrients absorbed by passive diffusion.

Topic Test 5.3: Answers

1. **True.** About one-third of absorbed glucose passes through the liver and is transported in the general circulation to others tissues.
2. **True.** The body has a limited capacity to store water-soluble vitamins and minerals. Once the body's needs are met, excess water-soluble vitamins and minerals are excreted in the urine.
3. **d.** Chylomicrons are made in the small intestine when dietary lipids are absorbed. They are composed mainly of triglyceride with smaller amounts of cholesterol and fat-soluble vitamins. Chylomicrons are transported first in the lymphatic system, then enter the general circulation via the left subclavian vein near the heart.
4. **c.** The liver, muscle, adipose, and brain are the tissues that capture the majority of dietary glucose.
5. Amino acids are water-soluble and, therefore, travel directly to the liver via the hepatic portal vein. Some amino acids are retained by the liver, while others pass through and are transported in the general circulation to other tissues. Excess amino acids not used for protein synthesis are transported back to the liver and metabolized for energy.
6. Both fructose and galactose are water-soluble nutrients and, consequently, are transported directly to the liver via the hepatic portal vein. Once in the liver, they are quickly removed from the blood and metabolized.

Chapter 6

Topic Test 6.1: Liver
True/False
1. The major blood vessel connecting the small intestine and liver is the hepatic portal vein.
2. After the body's protein needs are met, excess dietary amino acids are stored in the liver.

Multiple Choice
3. Dietary glucose entering the liver during the absorptive state is
   a. Broken down and used for energy
   b. Converted to glycogen for storage
   c. Converted to fatty acids and assembled into triglyceride
   d. All of the above
4. The liver receives dietary triglyceride
   a. Directly from the small intestine via the hepatic portal vein
   b. As chylomicron remnants
   c. As VLDL
   d. As micelles

Review Questions
5. In what ways does insulin regulate liver metabolism in the absorptive state?
6. What is the difference between chylomicrons and VLDL?

Topic Test 6.2: Muscle
True/False
1. Dietary amino acids are used primarily for energy in muscle.
2. The primary energy source for muscle in the absorptive state is fatty acids captured from circulating chylomicrons.

Multiple Choice
3. Muscle can store energy in the form of
   a. Glycogen
   b. Triglyceride
   c. Fatty acids
   d. All of the above
4. "Carbohydrate loading" refers to
   a. The ability of the brain to store glycogen
   b. Conversion of glucose to triglyceride in adipose
   c. Elevated blood glucose levels
   d. Maximizing the storage of glycogen in muscle

Review Questions
5. In what ways does insulin regulate muscle metabolism in the absorptive state?
6. How does muscle differ form the liver with regard to amino acid metabolism?

Topic Test 6.3: Adipose
True/False
1. The primary source of energy for adipose cells is blood glucose.
2. Adipose represents the body's largest potential reserve of energy.

Multiple Choice
3. The primary role of adipose tissues is to
   a. Store glycogen
   b. Store protein
   c. Store triglyceride
   d. All of the above
4. Adipose cells use the energy from glucose to
   a. Maintain body temperature
   b. Synthesize triglyceride
   c. Synthesize glycogen
   d. All of the above

Review Questions
5. In what ways does insulin regulate adipose metabolism in the absorptive state?
6. Explain why eating a diet rich in carbohydrate does not necessarily promote accumulation of triglyceride in adipose tissue.

Topic Test 6.4: Brain
True/False
1. Because of its critical function, the brain can use any energy source available in the body.
2. The brain lacks the ability to convert glucose to glycogen.

Multiple Choice
3. Under what condition can the brain adapt to alternative energy sources?
   a. In well-fed states
   b. Between meals
   c. When sleeping
   d. In starvation
4. The brain accounts for what percent of the body's total energy use?

a. 5%
b. 10%
c. 20%
d. 50%

Review Questions

5. With regard to energy needs, how is the brain different than liver, muscle, and adipose?
6. What do red blood cells and the brain have in common?

Topic Test 6.1: Answers

1. **True.** The hepatic portal vein is the only route through which water-soluble nutrients can enter the body after absorption.
2. **False.** The body does not store amino acids. Excess amino acids are used for energy in the liver.
3. **d.** The priority is to replenish the glycogen stores. However, any excess glucose will be used for energy or converted to fatty acids.
4. **b.** Dietary triglycerides enter the bloodstream as chylomicrons via the lymphatic system. After delivering most of the triglyceride to muscle and adipose, the chylomicron remnants (containing "leftover" triglyceride) are taken up by the liver.
5. Insulin promotes "building" processes in the liver such as glycogen synthesis (to store glucose), protein synthesis (to replenish blood proteins), and fatty acid and triglyceride synthesis (for transport to adipose for storage).
6. Both chylomicrons and VLDL are lipid–protein complexes that allow lipid (primarily triglyceride) to be carried in the bloodstream. The main difference is that chylomicrons originate in the small intestine and carry triglyceride absorbed from the diet, whereas VLDL carry triglyceride originating in the liver.

Topic Test 6.2: Answers

1. **False.** Amino acids are used to replenish muscle protein that was degraded since the last meal.
2. **False.** The primary energy source for muscle in the absorptive state is blood glucose.
3. **a.** Muscle cannot store fatty acids or triglyceride. Glycogen is the only storage form of energy in muscle.
4. **d.** Carbohydrate loading is the practice of consuming high-carbohydrate diets combined with specific exercises as a way of increasing glycogen storage in muscle. The diet/exercise regimen used for carbohydrate loading is usually begun several days before an athletic event.
5. Insulin promotes the uptake of glucose and amino acids from the blood. It also promotes the increase in glycogen and protein synthesis.
6. Both the liver and muscle use dietary amino acids to replenish proteins that were degraded since the last meal. After protein needs are fulfilled, both the liver and muscle can use excess amino acids for energy. However, only the liver can convert excess amino acids into fatty acids for triglyceride synthesis. The muscle lacks this ability and may release some of the excess amino acids back into the circulation.

Topic Test 6.3: Answers

1. **True.** Adipose does not use amino acids or fatty acids for energy under normal conditions.
2. **True.** Muscle and liver can also store energy as glycogen, but the capacity is limited in these tissues.
3. **c.** Adipose has an almost unlimited ability to store triglyceride. The triglycerides are made from fatty acids captured from circulating chylomicrons.
4. **b.** Glucose provides the energy for triglyceride assembly in adipose.
5. Insulin promotes the uptake of both glucose and fatty acids (from chylomicrons) into adipose cells. Insulin also stimulates triglyceride synthesis for storage.
6. Accumulation of body fat occurs only when total energy consumption exceeds the body's energy requirement. A diet rich in carbohydrate *per se* will not promote triglyceride accumulation in adipose unless the diet exceeds the body's energy needs.

Topic Test 6.4: Answers

1. **False.** Under normal circumstances, the brain uses only glucose as an energy source.
2. **True.** Consequently, the brain does not store glycogen (or any other energy source) and is completely dependent on the availability of blood glucose.
3. **d.** The brain will adapt to an alternative energy source in starvation or when dietary carbohydrate (glucose) is deficient.
4. **c.** The brain accounts for a significant portion of the body's basal metabolism.
5. Unlike most other tissues, the brain requires a constant supply of energy to maintain proper

body function. Furthermore, it can use only glucose for energy under normal conditions.
6. Red blood cells cannot store energy and rely on glucose as their sole source of energy.

Chapter 7

Topic Test 7.1: Liver

True/False
1. The hormone glucagon promotes gluconeogenesis.
2. Fatty acids are the only source of energy for the liver in fasting states.

Multiple Choice
3. The primary role of the liver in short-term fasting states is to
   a. Release glucose into the blood
   b. Release amino acids into the blood
   c. Release fatty acids into the blood
   d. Synthesize ketone bodies
4. The liver can make glucose from
   a. Fatty acids
   b. Amino acids
   c. Ketone bodies
   d. None of the above . . . the liver cannot make glucose

Review Questions
5. Explain why the liver does not use glucose for energy in short- or long-term fasting states.
6. What is the primary role of the liver in long-term fasting states?

Topic Test 7.2:   Muscle

True/False
1. Muscle glycogen is a major source of blood glucose in long-term fasting states.
2. "Muscle sparing" refers to the uptake and utilization of ketone bodies by muscle.

Multiple Choice
3. Which of the following is NOT used as an energy source in muscle?
   a. Glucose
   b. Fatty acids
   c. Amino acids
   d. Ketone bodies

4. Muscle activity accounts for about _____ of the body's total energy use.
   a. One-third
   b. One-half
   c. Two-thirds
   d. Three-fourths

Review Questions
5. What changes occur in muscle in short-term versus long-term fasting states?
6. What metabolic events in muscle are controlled by glucagon?

Topic Test 7.3: Adipose

True/False
1. The concentration of fatty acids in the blood significantly increases in long-term fasting states.
2. The hormone glucagon regulates the release of fatty acids from adipose.

Multiple Choice
3. As the duration of fasting increases, fatty acid release from adipose
   a. Gradually increases
   b. Gradually decreases
   c. Completely stops
   d. Does not change
4. Fatty acids are transported in the bloodstream
   a. As micelles
   b. As chylomicrons
   c. Bound to albumin
   d. Bound to VLDL

Review Questions
5. What is the main function of adipose in the body?
6. What nutrient is the primary source of energy for adipose cells in fasting states?

Topic Test 7.4: Brain

True/False
1. The brain can store limited amounts of glycogen for energy during fasting states.
2. The hormone glucagon promotes the uptake and use of ketone bodies by the brain.

Multiple Choice
3. In long-term fasting states, the brain can use which of the following for energy?
   a. Amino acids
   b. Fatty acids

c. Ketone bodies
d. All of the above
4. Beside the brain, what other tissue uses only glucose for energy?
   a. Pancreas
   b. Retina
   c. Adrenal glands
   d. Salivary glands

Review Questions

5. Describe how the liver, muscle, and adipose work together to keep the brain supplied with energy during fasting states.
6. How does ketone body use by the brain "spare muscle"?

Topic Test 7.1: Answers

1. True. Glucagon has the opposite action of insulin. Glucagon promotes glycogen breakdown to glucose, increases amino acid uptake into the liver, and promotes gluconeogenesis.
2. True. The liver uses glucose for energy only in the absorptive state when there is an abundance of dietary glucose.
3. a. The liver is the only organ that can maintain blood glucose levels within the normal range during short-term fasting states.
4. b. Amino acids from muscle protein are converted to glucose during short-term fasts via gluconeogenesis. To conserve muscle protein in long-term fasting states, gluconeogenesis decreases in prolonged situations of inadequate energy intake.
5. The liver conserves glucose by using fatty acids for energy. Liver glucose, whether from glycogen breakdown or gluconeogenesis, is the only source of glucose for maintaining blood levels.
6. The lack of dietary energy in long-term fasting states causes adipose to release fatty acids into the blood at an accelerated rate, flooding the liver with fatty acids for conversion to ketone bodies.

Topic Test 7.2: Answers

1. False. Muscle glycogen is used for energy only in muscle where it is stored. Muscle lacks the ability to release glucose into the blood.
2. False. Muscle sparing occurs in long-term fasting states when muscle no longer releases amino acids into the blood, thus retaining muscle mass.

3. c. Muscle uses amino acids only for building proteins.
4. a. Although somewhat dependent on the extent of physical activity, muscle accounts for about one-third of total energy expenditure in the body.
5. During short-term fasting states, muscle utilizes stored glycogen and fatty acids for energy. It also provides limited amounts of amino acids for liver to convert to glucose. When glycogen stores are depleted, muscle continues using fatty acids for energy and will gradually adapt to using ketone bodies.
6. Glucagon promotes reactions involved in energy utilization. In muscle these include glycogen conversion back to glucose, the breakdown of glucose for energy (glycolysis), and the breakdown of fatty acids for energy.

Topic Test 7.3: Answers

1. True. The flood of fatty acids entering the liver causes ketone body production to increase.
2. False. The hormones epinephrine and norepinephrine control the release of fatty acids from adipose.
3. a. The body gradually becomes more dependent on fatty acids from adipose as the primary energy source with increasing duration of fasting. Some fatty acids are used directly for energy, while others are converted to ketone bodies by the liver.
4. c. Upon release from adipose, fatty acids bind to the protein albumin for transport in the blood.
5. Adipose is the body's long-term energy reserve because of its ability to store large amounts of triglyceride. Secondarily, adipose acts as an insulator and as a cushion for internal organs.
6. Adipose cells use their own fatty acids for energy in fasting states. Blood glucose is also used for energy, but only in the absorptive state when blood glucose is abundant.

Topic Test 7.4: Answers

1. False. The brain cannot store glycogen and depends on a continual supply of glucose (or ketone bodies) from the blood.
2. False. Unlike other tissues, neither glucagon nor insulin is directly involved in brain metabolism.
3. c. The brain adapts to using ketone bodies when blood glucose levels decrease and blood ketone body levels increase. The brain will still use glucose if available.

4. **b.** In addition to retina, red blood cells and other nervous tissue depend on blood glucose as their sole source of energy.
5. In the absence of dietary nutrients, these tissues must work together to keep the brain functioning properly. In short-term fasting states, amino acids from muscle are converted to glucose by the liver. In long-term fasting states, fatty acids from adipose are converted to ketone bodies by the liver.
6. When the brain adapts to using ketone bodies, it becomes less dependent on glucose. In fasting states, blood glucose come from the conversion of amino acids, which sacrifices muscle protein.

Chapter 8

Topic Test 8.1: Energy Balance
True/False
1. Physical activity and muscle movement accounts for the majority of energy expended each day.
2. The US Department of Agriculture is the world's primary resource for finding the nutrient composition of food.

Multiple Choice
3. The basal metabolic rate for most adults can be estimated using the following equation:
   a. 1 kcal/kg of body weight per second
   b. 1 kcal/kg of body weight per minute
   c. 1 kcal/kg of body weight per hour
   d. 1 kcal/kg of body weight per day
4. All of the following are ways in which the body expends energy except
   a. Physical activity
   b. Storage of triglyceride
   c. Digestion of food
   d. Basal metabolism

Review Questions
5. What is basal metabolism?
6. Describe energy balance.

Topic Test 8.2: Body Fat—Too Much, Too Little
True/False
1. Leptin is a hormone made by fat cells that helps regulate appetite.

2. Too little body fat is associated with amenorrhea (absence of menstrual cycle) and an inability to sustain pregnancy.

Multiple Choice
3. Body mass index is
   a. A quantitative measure of disease
   b. A way of comparing weight relative to height
   c. An accurate measure of percent body fat
   d. Determined by skinfold measurements
4. Which of the following is not used in determining body fatness?
   a. Set point method
   b. Waist-to-hip ratio
   c. Underwater weighing
   d. Skinfold thickness

Review Questions
5. How were the "desirable" body weight tables first developed?
6. What is the "set point" theory?

Topic Test 8.3: Dieting vs. Weight Management
True/False
1. Weight management strategies are based on well-developed and carefully controlled energy restrictive diet plans.
2. Establishing a reasonable and healthy eating pattern can be achieved with the advice of a registered dietitian.

Multiple Choice
3. The goal of weight management programs is to
   a. Prevent further weight gain
   b. Establish normal eating patterns
   c. Increase physical activity
   d. All of the above
4. Short-term "diet" plans are usually successful at achieving weight loss because
   a. They cause the body to burn large amounts of stored fat
   b. They decrease appetite
   c. They cause the body to lose water
   d. They encourage increasing physical activity

Review Questions
5. Why do most "diets" fail?
6. What are the major differences between weight management and dieting?

Topic Test 8.1: Answers

1. F. Physical activity accounts for 20–30% of total energy expenditure in most adults. Although the percentage can be higher in athletes and very active people, basal metabolism uses most of the energy provided in the diet.
2. T. Several commercial databases are available for use of personal home computers, but most of them were developed from the USDA database.
3. c. Basal metabolism accounts for 60–70% of total energy expenditure in the average adult.
4. b. Storage of triglyceride represents a way in which the body captures energy for use at a later time.
5. Basal metabolism is the sum of all the involuntary activities that function in the body to support life. These functions include breathing, maintaining body temperature, and pumping blood.
6. Energy balance refers to the state in which body weight remains stable because the amount of energy consumed matches the amount used or expended by the body. Energy imbalance results in either body fat accumulation or loss of fat and muscle tissue.

Topic Test 8.2: Answers

1. T. As fat stores increase, the amount of leptin in the blood increases, which signals the brain to decrease appetite.
2. T. Too little body fat is also associated with a decreased ability of the immune system to ward off infection, as well as muscle wasting in individuals who suffer from chronic food shortages.
3. b. Body mass index is simply a way of converting two numbers (weight and height) into a single number. It provides no information about disease or **percent** body fat.
4. a. "Set point" is a theory—not a method—that helps explain how the body resists large changes in body fat.
5. The concept of "desirable" body weight was first developed by the life insurance industry. Using data from policy holders, body weight tables were established that corresponded to the lowest mortality rates. The health care industry later adopted similar tables for promoting public policy.
6. The set point theory is based on observations that the body generally resists large changes in body weight. When energy intake or physical activity change, the body's metabolism compensates to prevent significant changes in body fat. The set point theory helps explain why thin people have difficulty gaining body fat, while overweight people have difficulty losing excess body fat.

Topic Test 8.3: Answers

1. F. Weight management programs encourage the avoidance of diet plans and the establishment of reasonable eating patterns.
2. T. Registered dietitians are nutrition professionals who have completed a 4-year college degree in the nutrition area and who have met the established requirements set forth by the American Dietetic Association to certify them in providing nutrition counseling.
3. d. Unlike dieting, weight loss is not the goal of long-term weight management strategies.
4. c. The use of stored fat for energy is a relatively long-term metabolic process. Therefore, short-term weight loss is due mainly to losses of body water.
5. Energy-restrictive diets cause short-term weight loss, but have no secondary plan for keeping the weight off. Most dieters regain the lost weight because they do not change their eating behaviors after the dieting phase is over. In addition, short-term weight loss is mostly due to water loss, not fat loss.
6. Weight management is a long-term activity that occurs over a lifetime. It focuses on increasing physical activity and establishing reasonable eating patterns without dieting. Conversely, energy-restrictive dieting is a short-term activity that focuses entirely on weight loss. Dieting does not address physical activity and relies solely on decreasing energy intake for achieving weight loss goals.

Chapter 9

Topic Test 9.1: Coronary Heart Disease and Stroke

True/False

1. Coronary heart disease and stroke are really the same disease, except that they occur in different locations in the body.
2. Limiting sodium intake will cure hypertension in most people.

Multiple Choice

3. Which of the following is *not* a risk factor for CHD and stroke?
   a. Lack of exercise
   b. Iron deficiency
   c. Smoking
   d. Obesity
4. For a person with a slightly elevated serum cholesterol level of 230 mg/dL, the most appropriate treatment would be
   a. Prescription drugs
   b. Vitamin and mineral supplements
   c. Electroshock therapy
   d. Diet modification and exercise

Review Questions

5. How is it that someone could have atherosclerotic plaque but never experience a heart attack?
6. How is diet related to coronary heart disease and stroke?

Topic Test 9.2: Cancer

True/False

1. Cancer is the leading cause of death in the United States.
2. Nearly all foods contain potential carcinogens.

Multiple Choice

3. Which of the following is *not* a known dietary carcinogen?
   a. Charcoal broiled foods
   b. Polycyclic aromatic hydrocarbons
   c. Dietary fiber
   d. Nitrosamines
4. The growth of tissue containing cancer cells is called
   a. An oncogene
   b. An atheroma
   c. A plaque
   d. A neoplasm

Review Questions

5. What is cancer?
6. Describe how chemical carcinogens cause cancer.

Topic Test 9.3: Diabetes Mellitus

True/False

1. People with non-insulin-dependent diabetes mellitus must receive daily insulin injections for survival.
2. The American Diabetes Association promotes a special "diabetic diet" for all people with diabetes.

Multiple Choice

3. Which of the following is a strong risk factor for non-insulin-dependent diabetes mellitus?
   a. Low calcium intake
   b. Excess body fat
   c. High-protein diets
   d. High blood pressure
4. The onset of insulin-dependent diabetes mellitus is caused by
   a. Consumption of diets high in sugar
   b. Lack of exercise
   c. Autoimmune destruction of the cells that make insulin
   d. Elevated blood cholesterol

Review Questions

5. What are the differences between IDDM and NIDDM?
6. What are some of the long-term complications from hyperglycemia?

Topic Test 9.4: Osteoporosis

True/False

1. Smoking increases the risk of osteoporosis in women by decreasing estrogen levels in the body.
2. One of the best ways to prevent osteoporosis is to consume adequate amounts of both calcium and vitamin D.

Multiple Choice

3. The scientific term for "curvature of the spine" is
   a. Curvalosis
   b. Ketosis
   c. Kyphosis
   d. Trabeculosis
4. Which of the following is *not* a common type of calcium supplement?
   a. Multi-vitamin supplements
   b. Purified calcium compounds (such as calcium carbonate)
   c. Powdered oyster shell
   d. Bone meal tablets

Review Questions

5. What is the difference between Type I and Type II osteoporosis?
6. Why is osteoporosis called a "silent" disease?

Topic Test 9.1: Answers

1. **True.** Coronary heart disease is caused by plaque formation in the arteries that delivery blood to the heart, whereas stroke is due to the disease that develops in the arteries leading to the brain.
2. **False.** Hypertension is a complicated disease that is best treated by increasing physical activity and reducing excess body fat. Only about 15% of the population is sensitive to dietary sodium, so most people don't need to worry about salt or sodium intake.
3. **b.** Iron deficiency is associated with anemia (see Chapter 2), but it does not appear to play a role in atherosclerosis development.
4. **d.** The first approach to managing serum cholesterol levels should be adequate physical activity and a well-balanced diet rich in whole grains, fruits, and vegetables. Dietary supplements are usually unnecessary and prescription drugs should be used only in people with very high serum cholesterol who do not respond to diet and exercise.
5. Plaques build up inside arteries over many years without incident. It's only when they begin to restrict blood flow that they become problematic. A heart attack occurs when a plaque ruptures, causing a blood clot to form.
6. Many of the risk factors for CHD—including diabetes, hypertension, elevated serum cholesterol, and obesity—are strongly influenced by what we eat. In most cases, modifying one's diet and eliminating one or more of the risk factors can decrease the risk for CHD.

Topic Test 9.2: Answers

1. **True.** Cancer is responsible for about 23% of all deaths in the United States. Coronary heart disease accounts for about 20% of all deaths.
2. **True.** Although most foods contain natural chemicals that can initiate cancer, the body is equipped to "neutralize" and eliminate the vast majority of them, which is why most people will not develop cancer in their lifetime.
3. **c.** Dietary fiber is thought to reduce the risk of colorectal cancer by speeding the passage of potential carcinogens through the gastrointestinal tract.
4. **d.** Cancerous tissue is called a neoplasm. The common term is tumor.
5. Cancer is a group of related diseases characterized by the uncontrolled growth of cells originating from almost any tissue of the body.

The growth of cancer cells is caused by repeated exposure to substances in the environment (such as dietary carcinogens) or by internal factors (such as an inherited genetic mutation).
6. Exposure to a chemical carcinogen can eventually cause a permanent alteration to cellular DNA leading to the activation of a "cancer" gene called an oncogene. This results in transformation of the altered cells into malignant cancer cells that overtake and eventually kill off the native tissue from which they are growing.

Topic Test 9.3: Answers

1. **False.** Although some people with NIDDM can benefit from insulin injections (those with decreased insulin production by the pancreas), NIDDM is due mainly to insulin insensitivity in cells that take in glucose from the bloodstream such as muscle and adipose.
2. **False.** No single type of diet is appropriate for every person who suffers from diabetes. In general, people with both IDDM and NIDDM should follow the Food Guide Pyramid and current dietary guidelines to meet the body's nutrient requirements. Most diabetics need not exclude any single food item from their diet.
3. **b.** Obesity, advancing age, and physical inactivity are primary risk factors for NIDDM.
4. **c.** For unknown reasons, an autoimmune reaction destroys the beta-cells of the pancreas that make insulin. Most cases of IDDM occur before the age of 30.
5. The onset of IDDM usually occurs in childhood and results in the inability of the pancreas to make insulin. NIDDM usually occurs in overweight adults and is caused mainly by the inability of cells to respond to insulin. The pancreas is still able to produce insulin in NIDDM, although at a decreased rate.
6. Although the causes are not completely understood, hyperglycemia can cause blindness, kidney failure, nerve degeneration, and circulatory problems that may require amputation of the lower extremities. These complications can be largely avoided with proper treatment and management of blood glucose levels.

Topic Test 9.4: Answers

1. **True.** Estrogen promotes bone formation, although the exact biochemical mechanism is not fully understood.

2. **True.** Calcium is needed because it is the main structural component of bone. Vitamin D functions by increasing the absorption of dietary calcium in the small intestine. Deficiencies in either nutrient can result in osteoporosis.
3. **c.** Kyphosis, also called "Dowager's Hump," is caused by compression of the vertebrae due to the slow loss of bone calcium.
4. **a.** Multi-vitamin supplements provide vitamins, not minerals. Some dietary supplements contain both vitamins and minerals, but the word "mineral" must appear on the label.
5. Type I (or postmenopausal) osteoporosis occurs only in women as a result of declining estrogen levels. Type II osteoporosis occurs in both men and women as an inescapable result of aging. Type I and Type II are clinical definitions and it is often difficult to make a distinction between them in practice.
6. The loss of bone minerals often goes undetected because there are no symptoms in the early stages of the disease. Most people don't know they have osteoporosis until a bone fracture occurs.

Chapter 10

Topic Test 10.1: Pregnancy and Lactation
True/False
1. Scientifically developed infant formulas are better for newborn babies during the first few days because breast milk contains too much protein.
2. A woman's total energy intake needs to increase about 300 kilocalories per day during the second and third trimesters.

Multiple Choice
3. The recommended weight gain during pregnancy for normal weight woman is
   a. 35–45 pounds
   b. 25–35 pounds
   c. 15–25 pounds
   d. Less than 15 pounds
4. Two hormones involved in human milk production are
   a. Insulin and glucagon
   b. Lactase and sucrase

   c. Prolactin and oxytocin
   d. Trypsin and chymotrypsin

Review Questions
5. What are the major differences between infant formulas and breast milk?
6. Why should young woman who are not pregnant be concerned about consuming adequate amounts of folate?

Topic Test 10.2: From Infants to Teenagers
True/False
1. A mother who consumes a nutritionally poor diet can cause nutrient deficiencies in her breast-feeding infant.
2. The "extrusion reflex" refers to the process of human milk production and secretion.

Multiple Choice
3. Which of the following is *not* used in the manufacturing of infant formulas?
   a. Corn starch
   b. Vegetable oils
   c. Sugar (sucrose)
   d. Cows' milk
4. At what age is the growth rate of children the greatest?
   a. 6 months
   b. 2 years
   c. 6 years
   d. 12 years

Review Questions
5. When should solid foods be introduced into an infant's diet?
6. Why is it important to chart the growth pattern of growing children?

Topic Test 10.3: The Adult Years
True/False
1. Older adults are at increased risk for NIDDM diabetes mellitus because insulin sensitivity diminishes with age.
2. During the past 20 years, life expectancy in the United States has remained about the same.

Multiple Choice
3. What physiological change is *not* likely to affect the nutritional status of older adults?

a. Excess body fat accumulation
b. Impaired vision
c. Hair loss
d. Dental problems
4. Which of the following is most likely to be deficient in the diet of older adults?
   a. Fat
   b. Carbohydrate
   c. Vitamin C
   d. Calcium

Review Questions

5. Define aging.
6. Why is dehydration a common problem among the elderly?

Topic Test 10.1: Answer

1. **False.** Breast milk is the ideal food for infants of any age. It contains the perfect proportion of nutrients to allow babies to thrive. Milk produced during the first few days after childbirth is called "colostrum" and actually contains a higher proportion of protein than mature milk.
2. **True.** Pregnant women need to consume more essential nutrients and total energy to support the growth of a developing fetus. Total energy consumption generally needs to increase 300 kilocalories per day, but only during the second and third trimester when fetal growth is greatest.
3. **b.** Normal weight women should gain 25–35 pounds during pregnancy. Women who are underweight (BMI < 19.8) at the beginning of pregnancy need to gain more, while women who are overweight (BMI > 26.0) at the beginning of pregnancy should gain less.
4. **c.** The suckling of an infant causes the release of prolactin by the pituitary gland, which stimulates milk production. Oxytocin, also released by the pituitary gland, causes the milk to move from its storage lobes to the nipple in a process known as the let-down reflex.
5. In addition to the major nutrients, breast milk contains digestive enzymes, hormones, growth factors, antibodies, and several other beneficial substances that are not present in infant formulas. Most infant formulas are based on either cows' milk or soy protein, so the types of proteins present in formulas provide a different proportion of amino acids than that found in breast milk. Formulas are also made with vegetable oils, which contain a different proportion of fatty acids than breast milk.
6. Folate deficiency during pregnancy can cause neural tube defects because of its role during nerve cell development. The most critical period of development is during the first few weeks of pregnancy when many women are unaware they are pregnant. Therefore, all women of child-bearing age who are capable of becoming pregnant should consume a folate-adequate diet and consider taking a folate supplement.

Topic Test 10.2: Answer

1. **True.** Breast-feeding infants are completely dependent on mother's milk as their sole source of nutrients. All of the nutrients that are essential to the mother are essential to the infant as well. Consequently, nutrient deficiencies can easily develop in infants if the mother is consuming an insufficient diet.
2. **False.** The extrusion reflex refers to a protective mechanism in infants where the tongue is thrust forward to prevent any non-liquid objects from entering the mouth. Attempting to feed solid foods too early will cause the extrusion reflex.
3. **a.** The carbohydrates found in infant formulas are primarily simple sugars (lactose, sucrose, and/or corn syrups). The immature gastrointestinal tract of infants is ill prepared to handle complex carbohydrates.
4. **a.** Growth rate is greatest during the first few months of life; body weight will triple by 1 year of age. A second growth spurt occurs between puberty and adulthood, but the rate of growth is less than during infancy.
5. The American Academy of Pediatrics recommends that solid foods can be introduced between the age of 4 and 6 months, depending on when the infant is physically ready to receive them. Indicators of readiness include the ability to sit up, how well the infant can control head movement, the development of the gastrointestinal tract, and a diminishing extrusion reflex.
6. Following the growth pattern of children serves as an indicator of nutritional health. In healthy children, the growth pattern is more informative than the absolute weight. Growth patterns that are inconsistent with established growth curves should be a warning that nutrient deficiencies are present or that body fat accumulation is excessive.

Topic Test 10.3: Answer

1. **True.** Both insulin sensitivity in target tissues and insulin production by the pancreas diminish

with age. Consequently, blood glucose levels tend to increase, particularly in overweight individuals.

2. **False.** Life expectancy in the United States has increased throughout the past century and will likely rise in the future.

3. **c.** While hair loss per se does not affect nutritional status, certain nutrient deficiencies and medications can cause hair loss.

4. **d.** In addition to calcium, most older adults consume below the recommended amount of folate, vitamin D, vitamin E, magnesium, zinc, and total energy.

5. Aging is the natural progression of biological systems that is characterized by growth and change. Aging begins at conception and continues throughout life.

6. As people age, the sensation of thirst diminishes. Older adults usually need to drink fluids on a schedule rather than depending on their thirst response. Appetite decreases with age, so the intake of water present in food also decreases. The current recommendation for older adults is to consume the equivalent of 8 glasses of water per day.

Chapter 11

Topic Test 11.1: Food Choices

True/False

1. One of the strongest influences on food choice is taste.
2. The human brain instinctively knows what foods are needed to maintain good health.

Multiple Choice

3. Which of the following factors influencing our food choices has grown in importance during the past decade?
   a. Convenience
   b. Religious beliefs
   c. Level of education
   d. Cost

4. Which of the following is *not* a personal influence affecting our food choices?
   a. Habits
   b. Cultural traditions
   c. Perceived health beliefs
   d. Level of education

Review Questions

5. When a person must make dietary changes, why are small changes usually more successful over the long-run?
6. What do you consider to be the predominate factor affecting your food choices? And why?

Topic Test 11.2: To Eat Or Not to Eat

True/False

1. Eating in response to appetite rather than hunger can lead to overeating.
2. The part of the brain that regulates hunger and satiety is the hypothalamus.

Multiple Choice

3. Which of the following is related to appetite?
   a. Physical need to eat
   b. Feeling full and satisfied
   c. Headache, weakness, and stomach pains
   d. Choosing your favorite food

4. Which of the following is *not* likely to increase satiety?
   a. Elevated blood glucose levels
   b. Stomach expansion
   c. Decreased blood amino acids
   d. Elevated blood triglyceride levels

Review Questions

5. What is the difference between hunger and appetite?
6. Provide some examples of how our eating habits are influenced by appetite.

Topic Test 11.3: Eating Disorders

True/False

1. Eating disorders are seen mainly in females.
2. If you see someone who is extremely obese, you can assume they have binge-eating disorder.

Multiple Choice

3. Refusal to eat is the hallmark of which eating disorder?
   a. Binge-eating disorder
   b. Bulimia nervosa
   c. Anorexia nervosa
   d. Eating disorders not otherwise specified

4. Which of the following can help prevent eating disorders?
   a. Changing society's emphasis on thinness to be more realistic

b. Working with coaches to promote realistic weight expectations in athletes
c. Learning to separate food from our emotions
d. All of the above

Review Questions

5. Describe the cycle of events that define bulimia nervosa.
6. Why are eating disorders seen mainly in economically developed Western societies?

Topic Test 11.1: Answers

1. **True.** Few people routinely eat foods they dislike. Studies have shown that most people choose foods because they taste good.
2. **False.** While humans may have a genetic predisposition for certain foods, we do not have a built-in sensor that "tells" us what to eat to meet the body's nutrient needs. Rather, our food choices are driven mainly by external influences.
3. **a.** In general, people living in developed societies are preparing fewer meals in the home. Consequently, they have increased their consumption of pre-cooked, pre-packaged, and frozen foods. The sale of "fast foods" has also increased over the last few years.
4. **b.** Many cultural influences affect what we eat, including our traditions, religious beliefs, and what we deem to be acceptable.
5. Dietary changes are generally more successful when a person can continue eating the foods they enjoy. Small changes are less disruptive to a person's regular eating habits and, therefore, will be easier to maintain in the long term.
6. As you formulate your answer, consider all the personal, cultural, and practical influences that affect your food choices.

Topic Test 11.2: Answers

1. **True.** Because appetite is our psychological desire to eat, many people will eat even when they are not hungry. Learning to follow your body's hunger and satiety sensations can sometimes help people who are trying to control their food intake as part of an overall weight management program.
2. **True.** The hypothalamus responds to chemical signals and nerve impulses as it regulates both hunger and satiety sensations.
3. **d.** Unlike hunger and satiety, which are controlled by internal physical mechanisms, appetite is controlled by psychological cues. The desire to eat your favorite food can occur even when your stomach is full.
4. **c.** Satiety is initiated after a meal when the amount of blood amino acids, glucose, and triglycerides are elevated. Decreased amounts of blood amino acids are more likely to cause hunger sensations.
5. Hunger is our physical need to eat and is driven by internal body mechanisms. Hunger is associated with unpleasant physical sensations such as headache and stomach pains. Appetite is our psychological desire to eat and is triggered by external influences. Appetite is associated with the pleasurable aspects of eating and tends to guide our food choices.
6. Choosing a favorite food; eating at a certain time of day even when not hungry; desiring a food after seeing an advertisement; filling your plate regardless of its size; continuing to eat after feeling full.

Topic Test 11.3: Answers

1. **True.** Females, particularly young females, tend to feel greater pressure than males to be thin. Eating disorders in males are seen mainly in athletes (including wrestlers, weight lifters, jockeys, distance runners, and dancers).
2. **False.** A person can be considerably overweight and not have a binge-eating disorder. Obesity is caused by an energy imbalance and not necessarily by a psychological disorder. Diagnosis of binge-eating disorder is based upon the diagnostic criteria established for that disorder.
3. **c.** Although not a specific diagnostic criterion, refusal to eat adequate amounts of foods is driven by an intense fear of gaining weight or becoming fat. Individuals with anorexia nervosa see themselves as fat even when they are dangerously underweight.
4. **d.** Any strategy that will reduce expectations to be unrealistically thin will help to reduce the incidence of eating disorders.
5. Bulimia nervosa is characterized as bingeing in a short period of time, followed by purging. These events are then following by dieting or fasting. The bingeing/purging/dieting cycle can occur frequently over many years.
6. Western societies have, in general, created an unrealistic view of what a healthy, beautiful body should look like by promoting a certain body image through the media and entertainment

industry. Unfortunately, that view is overly thin and virtually impossible for most people to attain. The social pressure to look "thin and beautiful" is a major contributing factor to psychological eating disorders.

Chapter 12

Topic Test 12.1: From Research to Newspapers to Public Policy

True/False
1. Dietary recommendations for the public are usually published each time a new discovery is made in a research study.
2. It was discovered through scientific research that the outer hull of rice contains a toxic substance that causes gastrointestinal disorders and skin rash.

Multiple Choice
3. The scientific method *requires* which of the following?
   a. Development of a dietary recommendation
   b. Formulation of a testable hypothesis
   c. Publication of research results on the internet
   d. Development of a news release for the media
4. Consumers get most of their nutrition information from
   a. Newspaper articles
   b. Women's magazines
   c. Television news broadcasts
   d. All of the above

Review Questions
5. Briefly describe the scientific method.
6. Why do scientists use statistics when analyzing results from their research studies?

Topic Test 12.2: Understanding Disease Risk

True/False
1. The branch of science that focuses on diet and disease relationships is called epidemiology.
2. An individual can easily assess his or her personal risk of disease using data from epidemiologic studies.

Multiple Choice
3. Which of the following is *not* commonly used to assess food consumption?
   a. Food frequency questionnaire
   b. Food diary
   c. Meal plate count
   d. 24-hour recall
4. The epidemiologic term used to describe what people eat is
   a. Utilization
   b. Prevalence
   c. Association
   d. Exposure

Review Questions
5. How would you describe "disease risk"?
6. What are the two types of measurements needed for calculating disease risk?

Topic Test 12.3: Interpreting Nutrition Information

True/False
1. Health claims must be reviewed by a scientific panel before they can be used in advertising.
2. The primary motive of advertising is the desire to improve the health of consumers.

Multiple Choice
3. The deceptive promotion of nutrition related products, treatments, or plans solely for financial gain is known as
   a. Blasphemy
   b. Skullduggery
   c. Quackery
   d. Debauchery
4. Of the following, which is the most important question you could ask when trying to determine the reliability of nutrition information?
   a. "Does someone stand to profit by providing the information?"
   b. "How recent was the information published?"
   c. "Is the information available on the internet?"
   d. "Is an address and telephone number provided with the information?"

Review Questions
5. List all of the possible sources of nutrition information you can think of. Which source is *your* primary source of information?
6. Why has it become necessary for each of us to have a system of evaluation regarding nutrition information?

Topic Test 12.1: Answers

1. **False.** Dietary recommendations for the public are usually made after a critical mass of information has been gathered and carefully reviewed by public health officials and other experts.
2. **False.** The outer hull of rice contains niacin, an essential nutrient required for normal growth and good health.
3. **b.** While each of the answers are associated with research, the only requirement of the scientific method is the formulation of a testable hypothesis (which will then be tested by experimentation).
4. **d.** Few consumers get nutrition information from scientific journals in which the original research was published. Most people rely on media sources and the internet for their nutrition information.
5. The scientific method is a systematic approach to better understanding natural phenomena. It involves proposing hypotheses that might explain observations, then conducting experiments to see if the hypothesis will be accepted or rejected. The scientific method is a "process of elimination" that gradually paints a picture of explanation one step at a time.
6. Analyzing data using statistics helps researchers quantify the amount of error that exists in their studies. Putting their study results into mathematical terms is thought to increase the validity of the research as well as the confidence in drawing conclusions.

Topic Test 12.2: Answers

1. **True.** More specifically, epidemiology deals the various dietary (and other) factors associated with the frequency and distribution of diseases in a population.
2. **False.** Disease risk is determined using data from large numbers of people and, therefore, has limited application to single individuals.
3. **c.** The 24-hour recall and the food diary require subjects to estimate portion size, whereas the food frequency questionnaire includes a list of foods commonly consumed in the population and asks subjects to indicate how frequently those foods are consumed in their overall diet.
4. **d.** "Exposure" is also used in other types of epidemiologic studies that examine determinants of disease other than diet (e.g., asbestos and lung cancer).

5. Disease risk is a mathematical expression of the relationship between a dietary component and the occurrence of disease. Epidemiologic studies with large numbers of people are needed to generate the data used in calculating disease risk.
6. Measuring disease risk requires the ability to accurately measure what people eat and the ability to document what diseases they develop.

Topic Test 12.3: Answers

1. **False.** Some sources of information, such as the information on Nutrition Facts panels, are required to conform to government standards of accuracy. However, the vast majority of information used to sell products and dietary plans is not required to meet any standard of truth before it is made available to the public.
2. **False.** While it is conceivable that some manufacturers and distributors of health-related products are concerned about the welfare of consumers, the primary motive is money.
3. **c.** The term "quackery" comes from the days when traveling salesmen would set up displays in the town square and "quack" about their salves, tonics, and elixirs. These miracle health products were touted as curing virtually any ailment known to man.
4. **a.** When the sole motive is financial gain, the chance of encountering fraudulent health claims greatly increases. Although the internet contains vast amounts of bogus and misleading "facts" about nutrition, many reputable organizations provide accurate nutrition information on the internet. Simply providing an address and phone number does not guarantee that additional information will be any more reliable.
5. Possible sources of nutrition information include: newspapers, magazines, textbooks, school teachers, television, radio, research journals, advertisements, infomercials, food labels, government reports, the internet, friends, family members, store employees, physicians, pharmacists, dietitians, and other health care professionals.
6. Nutrition information is not subject to any standard of truth and there are few laws regulating how nutrition information is dispensed to the public. Consequently, there is a great opportunity for fraudulent information to find its way into society. Judging the accuracy and reliability of nutrition information has become necessary to protect both our health and pocketbooks.

Chapter 13

Topic Test 13.1: Food Technology

True/False

1. Cold temperature storage is not a very effective way to preserve food.
2. The term "shelf life" refers to the length of time foods can be stored without spoiling.

Multiple Choice

3. Which of the following is not a function of food additives?
   a. Enhance the flavor, color, and texture
   b. Enhance the nutritional quality of food
   c. Increase the temperature of food
   d. Prevent growth of microorganisms
4. The government agency that oversees the use of food additives in the United States is
   a. The National Institutes of Health
   b. The US Department of Agriculture
   c. The Food and Drug Administration
   d. The Centers for Disease Control and Prevention

Review Questions

5. Why are many foods treated with high temperature during processing?
6. What do the food processing terms "fortification" and "enrichment" mean?

Topic Test 13.2: Food-Borne Illness

True/False

1. "Food-borne infection" refers to the ingestion of small amounts of chemical toxins.
2. Many people who experience a food-borne illness mistakenly believe they have the flu.

Multiple Choice

3. Food-borne illness can be minimized by each of the following *except*
   a. Wash hands and cooking utensils frequently
   b. Select only the freshest foods when shopping
   c. Store all foods at room temperature
   d. Cook foods thoroughly
4. Cross-contamination refers to
   a. The production of toxins by bacteria
   b. The transfer of microorganisms from one food to another
   c. The improper use of chemical pesticides
   d. The presence of parasites in fruits and vegetables

Review Questions

5. Describe the HACCP approach to food safety.
6. What is a pathogen?

Topic Test 13.3: Food Labeling

True/False

1. The law requires that fresh meat, fish, and poultry be individually labeled with the Nutrition Facts panel.
2. The % Daily Value for vitamin A and vitamin C is the only required information regarding vitamins on the Nutrition Facts panel.

Multiple Choice

3. Which of the following is *not* a labeling requirement on food products having more than one ingredient?
   a. A list of the ingredients
   b. The name and address of the manufacturer, packager, or distributor
   c. The product's nutrient content
   d. A statement of the product's health benefits
4. Irradiation
   a. Preserves foods by preventing oxidation
   b. Is not very useful for fruits and vegetables
   c. Can make certain foods radioactive
   d. Is a safe and effective way to preserve food

Review Questions

5. Why were food labeling laws developed in the United States?
6. What is the % Daily Value?

Topic Test 13.4: Functional Foods

True/False

1. Federal law allows manufacturers of functional foods to make specific health claims on the product label.
2. The health benefits of functional foods have been well documented in hundreds of scientific studies.

Multiple Choice

3. Which of the following is *not* a phytochemical used in the manufacture of functional foods?
   a. Flavonoids
   b. Carotenoids
   c. Phytosterols
   d. Cholesterol
4. Which of the following is *not* an example of a functional food?
   a. Beef patty made with added soy protein
   b. Vegetarian lasagna made with spinach and zucchini
   c. Margarine made with phytosterols
   d. Carbonated soft drink containing ginseng and echinacea

Review Questions

5. What is the difference between a functional food and a nutraceutical?
6. How do we distinguish between a functional food and a drug?

Topic Test 13.1: Answers

1. **False.** Cold temperature inhibits the growth of microorganisms, which allows food companies to make a wide variety of refrigerated and frozen food products.
2. **True.** Extending the shelf life of foods is a primary concern of the food industry.
3. **c.** No food additive can increase the temperature of food—only heat or microwaves can do that.
4. **c.** The FDA grants approval for using a food additive only after extensive research on its safety and efficacy.
5. The main cause of food spoilage and food-related illness is the growth of microorganisms. Treating foods to high temperature kills the microorganisms, thus extending the foods' shelf life and making them safer to consume.
6. Fortification is a general term describing the addition of nutrients to foods. Enrichment is a type of fortification in which the nutrients added to foods are intended to replace those lost during processing. The addition of water-soluble vitamins to refined flour is a prime example of enrichment.

Topic Test 13.2: Answers

1. **False.** Food-borne infection is caused by the ingestion of relatively large numbers of bacteria or other living microorganism that grow in the gastrointestinal tract.
2. **True.** The symptoms of food-borne illness are similar to influenza and include diarrhea, headache, and nausea.
3. **c.** Fresh meats, fruits, vegetables, and other perishable foods should be stored in the refrigerator or freezer. Cooked foods should also be stored at cold temperatures.
4. **b.** Cross-contamination can be avoided by cleaning kitchen surfaces and washing hands and utensils after every step during food preparation.
5. Hazard Analysis Critical Control Point (HACCP) is a food safety system that focuses on identifying and preventing contamination during processing that could cause food-borne illness. Each processor and manufacturer is required to set up their own HACCP plan so that critical steps in the food handling process can be identified and monitored.
6. A pathogen is any microorganisms capable of causing illness when ingested. Pathogens include bacteria, viruses, molds, and parasites.

Topic Test 13.3: Answers

1. **False.** Fresh fruits, vegetables, meat, fish, and poultry do not have to be individually labeled, although information regarding their nutrient content can be found in most grocery stores.
2. **True.** Information regarding all other vitamins is voluntary.
3. **d.** Claims regarding the product's nutritive or health properties are voluntary.
4. **d.** The major obstacle facing the use of irradiation is consumer skepticism. Many of the public's concerns are similar to those raised in the 1960s when microwave ovens were first being sold.
5. Food labeling laws were created to give consumers more detailed information about the nutrient content of food products for the purpose of making food purchasing decisions in planning their diets wisely.
6. The % Daily Value for a single nutrient is the amount per serving compared to a daily reference amount for that nutrient, based on a 2,000-Calorie diet.

Topic Test 13.4: Answers

1. **True.** Health claims are allowed, but they must be accompanied by: "This statement has not been evaluated by the Food and Drug Administration.

This product is not intended to diagnose, treat, cure or prevent any disease."

2. **False.** While food has been used as a therapeutic agent for centuries, very little scientific evidence exists regarding the long-term health benefits of functional foods.

3. **d.** Cholesterol is a substance found only in animal foods. Consumption of cholesterol is believed to increase the risk of heart disease in some people.

4. **b.** From a food industry perspective, it is unlikely that vegetarian lasagna would be classified as a functional food. Although it is made with vegetables (in this case spinach and zucchini), the added vegetables are usually not to be considered "nutraceuticals" to the same extent as the other isolated phytochemicals.

5. "Functional foods" are products that contain substances believed to provide health benefits beyond the basic nutrient requirements of the body. The term "nutraceutical" refers to the specific substance added to functional foods.

6. "Drugs" are currently defined as substances that "diagnosis, treat, prevent, cure, or mitigate disease." While this is how many people view functional foods, the laws that govern the manufacture and sale of drugs and foods are separate. And even though drugs and functional foods may contain the same added chemical, functional foods are not subject to the same level of testing and scrutiny regarding their safety.

Chapter 14

Topic Test 14.1: Physical Activity

True/False

1. The Dietary Guidelines for Americans recommend that people "Aim for Fitness" by engaging in some form of moderate physical activity every day.

2. During short-duration, high-intensity activities, amino acids (from protein breakdown) provide the major source of energy for muscle movement.

Multiple Choice

3. Which of the following is *not* true about lactic acid?
   a. It accumulates in muscle when oxygen supply is low

b. It can be used by the liver to make glucose
   c. It is a product of aerobic metabolism
   d. It causes painful muscles

4. Regular exercise is associated with each of the following *except*:
   a. Reduces risk of obesity
   b. Improves sleep
   c. Reduces risk of heart disease
   d. Increases resting heart rate

Review Questions

5. What role does phosphocreatine play in muscle movement?

6. Why does low-intensity, long-duration exercise cause muscle to use a greater proportion of fatty acids than glucose for energy?

Topic Test 14.2: The Concept of Optimal Health

True/False

1. "Optimal health" is a well-defined, easily measured physical condition.

2. Ayurveda may be described as a way of life that focuses on the proper balance of the senses, mind, body, and soul.

Multiple Choice

3. In Traditional Chinese Medicine, a practitioner will feel the pulse of a patient
   a. To measure percent body fat
   b. To assess subtle imbalances in the patient's health
   c. To determine blood glucose concentration
   d. To measure blood pressure

4. Achieving optimal health requires a person to recognize that
   a. Optimal health cannot be measured by traditional scientific methods
   b. Optimal health is a state of wellness unique to every individual
   c. Optimal health includes both physical and mental states of well being
   d. All of the above

Review Questions

5. What is the major limitation of biomedical science in addressing the concept the optimal health?

6. What is Traditional Chinese Medicine?

Topic Test 14.3: Information Resources

True/False

1. For the most in-depth and accurate information regarding diet and nutrition, physicians are always the best resource.
2. There are no specific laws governing the use of the title "nutritionist."

Multiple Choice

3. Which of the following is least likely to be a reliable source of accurate nutrition information?
   a. "Herbal Life" Products Catalog
   b. The Mayo Clinic Health Information website
   c. The National Center for Complementary and Alternative Medicine
   d. The American Dietetic Association
4. To become a registered dietitian, each of the following requirements must be fulfilled *except*:
   a. Pass the national ADA registration examination
   b. Earn a bachelor's degree and satisfy specific coursework requirements
   c. Complete a supervised practice program (internship)
   d. Have 2 years' experience in restaurant foodservice

Review Questions

5. What careers are available to qualified individuals in the nutrition field?
6. List some of the courses a person must take to be eligible for the ADA registration examination.

Topic Test 14.1: Answers

1. **True.** The guidelines recommend at least 30 minutes daily for adults and 60 minutes daily for children.
2. **False.** Glucose is the primary fuel during short-duration, high-intensity exercise. The only time significant amounts of amino acids are used for muscle energy is during long-duration activities of moderate to high intensity such as marathon running.
3. **c.** Lactic acid is a product of anaerobic metabolism. It is made from the incomplete breakdown of glucose when oxygen is not available.
4. **d.** Regular exercise improves oxygen carrying capacity of the cardiovascular system by strengthening the heart muscle. The result is a lowering of the resting heart rate.
5. Muscle movement depends on adequate

amounts of ATP. Phosphocreatine is a high-energy molecule in muscle cells that can quickly transfer energy to ATP. Although there is about five times more phosphocreatine than ATP in resting muscle, phosphocreatine cannot be used directly for energy. Phosphocreatine (and ATP) can be regenerated from glucose, fatty acids, and amino acids.
6. Low-intensity, long-duration exercise uses fatty acids from adipose tissue as a way of conserving muscle glycogen for times when very rapid, high-intensity muscle movement is required. Because glucose is stored in muscle, it can be thought of as an immediate energy source for muscle, whereas fatty acids are a more long-term energy source.

Topic Test 14.2: Answers

1. **False.** While there is no single definition of optimal health, it clearly cannot be described solely on the basis of physical measurements. It may be best described as an optimal state of physical and mental wellness that is unique to each individual.
2. **True.** Ayurveda has been a guiding principle and a way of life in India for more than 4,000 years.
3. **b.** Chinese pulse theory does not rely on quantifying physical indicators of health. Rather, it distinguishes the quality of the pulse that may be expressed in descriptive terms, such as hollow or soggy, for the purpose of detecting subtle imbalances before they manifest themselves as a clinical disease.
4. **d.** Although not easy to define, the concept of optimal health is based on the belief that all aspects of a person's well being must be in balance. This includes physical well being as well as mental and spiritual well being. Scientific measurements of physical well being are useful in assessing health, but they only provide one view of a person's total health.
5. Science is a system of inquiry that depends on objective, measurable outcomes. In this sense, scientific research is able to address only those aspects of health that are measurable, such as blood pressure or body weight. The concept of optimal health has few (if any) measurable indicators that the scientific method can address.
6. Traditional Chinese Medicine is an ancient system of health care that is based on principles of balance and countermeasures that strive to keep the body's opposing energies (called Yin and Yang) in balance and flowing properly

through the body's energy pathways (called meridians).

Topic Test 14.3: Answers

1. **Not always.** Many physicians are well trained in nutrition-related aspects of health, but only about one-fourth of all medical schools in the United States required even one course in nutrition.
2. **True.** The term "nutritionist" has no specific reference with regard to health organizations in the United States. Anyone can call themselves a nutritionist.
3. **a.** Any source of information that promotes the sale of a product is likely to contain biased information.
4. **d.** Taking specific courses in foodservice management is part of the coursework requirements for the RD credential, but having previous experience working in a restaurant is not a requirement.
5. Positions related to foodservice management, food production and preparation, and nutrition counseling are among the most popular for individuals with proper training in nutrition or dietetics. Many positions required applicants to have the RD credential. These positions can be found in hospitals, corporations, schools, and public health and volunteer agencies.
6. Food and nutrition sciences; foodservice systems management; business; economics; educational psychology; chemistry; biochemistry; microbiology; anatomy; physiology.

Index

Note: Page numbers in *italics* refer to Figures; those in **bold** to Tables